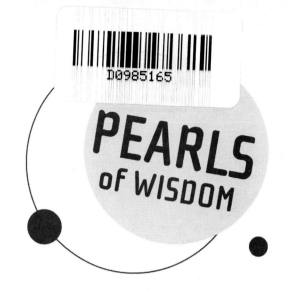

ACLS
(Advanced Cardiac Life Support)
REVIEW

Second Edition

Michael Zevitz
Scott H. Plantz
William G. Gossman

McGraw-Hill
Medical Publishing Division

New York Chicago San Francisco Lisbon London
Madrid Mexico City Milan New Delhi
San Juan Seoul Singapore
Sydney Toronto

The **McGraw·Hill** Companies

ACLS (Advanced Cardiac Life Support) Review, Second Edition

1 2 3 4 5 6 7 8 9 0 CUS/CUS 0 9 8 7 6 5

ISBN 0-07-146401-8

Notice

Medicine is an ever-changing science. As new research and clinical experience broaden our knowledge, changes in treatment and drug therapy are required. The authors and the publisher of this work have checked with sources believed to be reliable in their efforts to provide information that is complete and generally in accord with the standards accepted at the time of publication. However, in view of the possibility of human error or changes in medical sciences, neither the authors nor the publisher nor any other party who has been involved in the preparation or publication of this work warrants that the information contained herein is in every respect accurate or complete, and they disclaim all responsibility for any errors or omissions or for the results obtained from use of the information contained in this work. Readers are encouraged to confirm the information contained herein with other sources. For example and in particular, readers are advised to check the product information sheet included in the package of each drug they plan to administer to be certain that the information contained in this work is accurate and that changes have not been made in the recommended dose or in the contraindications for administration. This recommendation is of particular importance in connection with new or infrequently used drugs.

The editors were Catherine A. Johnson and Marsha Loeb.
The production supervisor was Phil Galea.
The cover designer was Handel Low.
Von Hoffmann Graphics was printer and binder.

This book is printed on acid-free paper.

Cataloging-in-Publication data for this title is on file at the Library of Congress.

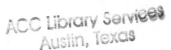

DEDICATION

To my parents, Norman and Dorothy, whose love and emphasis on my education was the rock on which my personal and professional life was founded and remains to this day.

Michael Zevitz

EDITORS

Michael Zevitz, M.D.
Assistant Professor of Medicine
Division of Cardiology
Chicago Medical School
Chicago, Illinois

Scott Plantz, M.D.
Associate Professor and Research Director
Department of Emergency Medicine
Mt. Sinai Medical Center
Chicago, Illinois

William Gossman, M.D.
Assistant Professor and EMS Director
Dept. of Emergency Medicine
Mt. Sinai Medical Center
Chicago, Illinois

CONTRIBUTING AUTHORS

Guy H. Haskell, Ph.D., NREMT-P
Associate Professor
Emergency Medical Services Education
Bloomington Hospital
Bloomington, Indiana

Lt. Robert C. Krause, EMT-P
Toledo Fire and Rescue
Toledo, Ohio

Diane M. Bourgeois, M.Ed., EMT-B
Emergency Medical Services Program
Quinsigamond Community College
Worcester, Massachusetts

Brandy DeBarge, EMT-D
Emergency Medical Services Program
Quinsigamond Community College
Worcester, Massachusetts

John Wypyszinski, EMT-B
Emergency Medical Services Program
Quinsigamond Community College
Worcester, Massachusetts

INTRODUCTION

Nothing in the world can take the place of persistence. Talent will not; nothing is more common than unsuccessful men with talent. Genius will not; unrewarded genius is almost a proverb. Education will not; the world is full of educated derelicts. Persistence and determination alone are omnipotent.
Calvin Coolidge

Congratulations! *ACLS Review: Pearls of Wisdom* will help you pass the Advanced Cardiac Life Support Course of the American Heart Association. This book's unique format differs from all other review and test preparation texts. Let us begin, then, with a few words on purpose, format, and use.

The primary intent of this book is to serve as a rapid review of ACLS principles and serve as a study aid to improve performance on the ACLS written and practical examinations. With this goal in mind, the text is written in rapid-fire, question/answer format. The student receives immediate gratification with a correct answer. Questions themselves often contain a "pearl" reinforced in association with the question/answer.

Additional hooks are often attached to the answer in various forms, including mnemonics, evoked visual imagery, repetition, and humor. Additional information not requested in the question may be included in the answer. The same information is often sought in several different questions. Emphasis has been placed on evoking both trivia and key facts that are easily overlooked, are quickly forgotten, and yet somehow always seem to appear on ACLS exams.

Many questions have answers without explanations. This is done to enhance ease of reading and rate of learning. Explanations often occur in a later question/answer. It may happen that upon reading an answer the reader may think - "Hmm, why is that?" or, "Are you sure?" If this happens to you, GO CHECK! Truly assimilating these disparate facts into a framework of knowledge absolutely requires further reading in the surrounding concepts. Information learned, as a response to seeking an answer to a particular question is much better retained than that passively read. Take advantage of this. Use *ACLS Review* with your ACLS text handy and open, or, if you are reviewing on train, plane, or camelback, mark questions for further investigation.

ACLS Review risks accuracy by aggressively pruning complex concepts down to the simplest kernel. The dynamic knowledge base and clinical practice of medicine is not like that! The information taken as "correct" is that indicated in the ACLS American Heart Association text. New research and practice occasionally deviates from that which likely represents the "right" answers for test purposes. In such cases we have selected the information that we believe is most likely "correct" for test purposes, which most closely conforms to the ACLS curriculum. This text is designed to maximize your score on a test. Refer to the ACLS text for further information and your mentors for direction on current practice.

ACLS Review is designed to be used, not just read. It is an interactive text. Use a 3x5 card and cover the answers; attempt all questions. A study method we strongly recommend is oral, group study, preferably over an extended meal or pitchers. The mechanics of this method are simple and no one ever appears stupid. One person holds *ACLS Review*, with answers covered, and reads the question. Each person, including the reader, says "Check!" when he or she has an answer in mind. After everyone has "checked" in, someone states his or her answer. If this answer is correct, on to the next one. If not, another person states his or her answer, or the answer can be read. Usually, the person who "checks" in first gets the first shot at stating the answer. If this person is being a smarty-pants answer-hog, then others can take turns. Try it--it's almost fun!

ACLS Review is also designed to be re-used several times to allow, dare we use the word, memorization. One co-editor (Plantz), a pessimist, suggests putting a check mark beside the question every time a question is missed. If you have two checks on re-use of *ACLS Review*, forget this question! You will get it wrong on the exam! Another suggestion is to place a check mark when the question is answered correctly once; skip all questions with check marks thereafter. Utilize whatever scheme you prefer.

We welcome your comments, suggestions and criticism. Great effort has been made to verify these questions and answers. There will be answers we have provided that are at variance with the answer you would prefer. Most often this is attributable to the variance between original source (previously discussed). Please make us aware of any errata you find. We hope to make continuous improvements in a second edition and would greatly appreciate any input with regard to format, organization, content, presentation, or about specific questions. We look forward to hearing from you.

Study hard and good luck!

M.Z., S.H.P., & W.G.G.

TABLE OF CONTENTS

PRE-TEST

○ **What is the treatment for the following rhythm in a stable patient with a heart rate of 180 beats per minute, blood pressure 120/80, and respiratory rate of 16?**

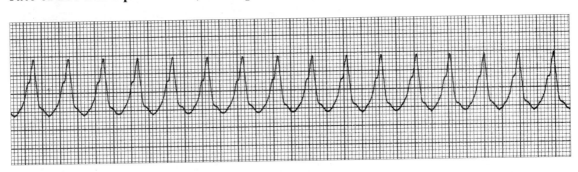

Stable ventricular tachycardia is treated with O2, IV, and monitor and administration of lidocaine at 1-1.5 mg/kg IV bolus. A repeat dose may be given at 0.5-0.75 mg/kg every 5 minutes to a maximum dose of 3 mg/kg.

○ **What are the possible causes of pulseless electrical activity?**

Acidosis, cardiac tamponade, tension pneumothorax, hypovolemia, hypoxia, hyperkalemia, hypothermia, pulmonary embolism, extensive acute myocardial infarction, and drug overdose (Most notably calcium channel blocker overdose).

○ **What is the following rhythm?**

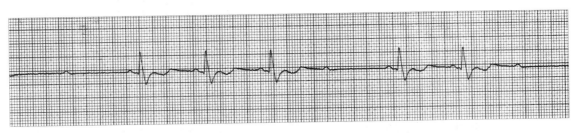

Second degree AV block, type II. Features include:
- Rate: atrial rate greater than ventricular rate
- Rhythm: atrial rhythm regular, ventricular rhythm irregular
- P waves: normal in size and configuration
- P-R interval: may be normal or prolonged, but constant for each conductive QRS
- QRS: greater than 0.10 seconds, intermittently absent

○ **What is the following rhythm?**

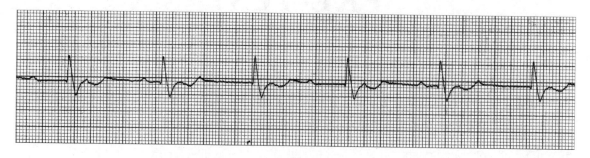

Complete heart block. Characteristics include:

- Rate: atrial rate greater than ventricular rate
- Rhythm: atrial rhythm is regular, ventricular rhythm is regular
- P waves: more frequent than QRS complexes
- P-R interval: the atria and ventricles beat independently of each other; there is no relationship between P and QRS complexes
- QRS: may be narrow or wide depending on location of the escape pacemaker; narrow is due to a junctional escape rhythm whereas wide is due to a ventricular escape rhythm

○ **What is the following rhythm?**

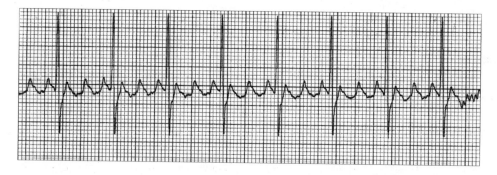

Atrial flutter.

○ **What is the following rhythm?**

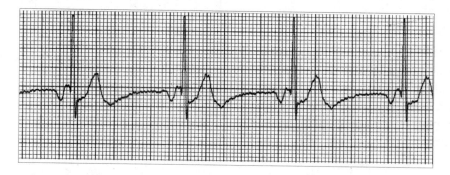

Junctional rhythm.
Key features include:

- Rate: 40-60 beats per minute
- Rhythm: atrial and ventricular rhythm regular
- P waves may occur before, during, or after the QRS, often inverted
- P-R interval: generally not measurable unless the P wave precedes the QRS
- QRS: 0.10 seconds or less

○ What is the most common cause of an accelerated junctional rhythm?

Digitalis toxicity

○ What is the following rhythm?

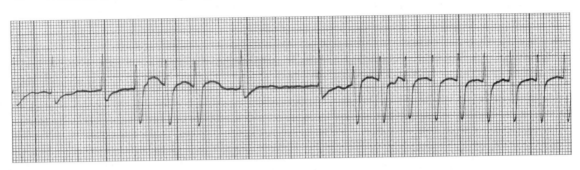

Atrial fibrillation with runs of ventricular tachycardia.

○ What are the ECG findings suspected in a patient with hyperkalemia?

K 6.5 to 7.5 mEq/L - prolonged P-R interval, widened QRS, decrease in P wave amplitude, tall-peaked T waves and ST segment depression or elevation.

K 7.5 to 8.5 mEq/L - wide QRS, further flattening of the P wave with widening, bundle branch blocks as well as AV blocks may occur.

K greater than 8.5 mEq/L - P wave is absent, very wide QRS, ventricular dysrhythmias including V-fib, V-tach, and asystole.

○ What are the causes of cardiac dysrhythmias?

Disturbances in conductivity, such as with Wolff-Parkinson-White syndrome or AV block and disturbances in automaticity, such as premature atrial, junctional or ventricular complexes, atrial or ventricular tachycardia, sinus bradycardia, and sinus tachycardia.

○ A conduction defect above the level of the His bundle will result in _____.

Changes in P wave and P-R interval.

○   **Conduction defects at or below the level of the His bundle will result in _____.**

Conduction problems involving the QRS complex with QRS widening.

○   **What is supraventricular tachycardia?**

It is a nonspecific dysrhythmia that cannot be individually distinguished due to its high rate. SVT is characterized by a narrow QRS complex in which P waves often cannot be distinguished from the preceding T wave.

○   **What are the possible causes of Torsades de Pointes?**

Anorexia, bulimia, electrolyte abnormalities, and drug-induced; typically by tricyclic antidepressants.   Also, antidysrhythmics, including procainamide, flecainide, and quinidine, antibiotics, such as erythromycin, and antihistamines, such as terfenadine.

○   **What are the characteristic features of supraventricular tachycardia?**

A slightly irregular ventricular rhythm, narrow QRS complex, and P waves often indistinguishable from preceding T waves.

○   **T/F: The QRS complex may be narrow or wide in third degree (complete) AV block.**

True. The QRS complex will be narrow if a junctional escape rhythm is present and wide if a ventricular escape rhythm is present.

○   **What is the differential diagnosis of third degree (complete) AV block?**

Digitalis toxicity, ischemia, congenital abnormalities, rheumatic fever, acute inferior wall MI, and conduction system disease.

○   **What is the effect of hypomagnesemia on an ECG?**

Prolonged P-R interval, ST segment depression, and flattened T waves.

○   **How do you characterize multifocal atrial tachycardia?**

- Rate: Greater than 100 beats per minute
- Rhythm: Atrial and ventricular rhythms are irregular
- P-R interval: may be normal or variable
- P waves: polymorphic (multiple types of P wave configuration)
- QRS: normal

❍ **What is Wolff-Parkinson-White syndrome?**

It is the most common type of pre-excitation syndrome in which a bundle of working myocardial tissue forms a connection outside the normal atrioventricular conductive pathway.

❍ **What are the common causes of second degree AV block type I?**

Digitalis toxicity, drugs such as verapamil and propranolol, rheumatic fever, inferior wall MI, and increased parasympathetic tone.

❍ **What is the following rhythm?**

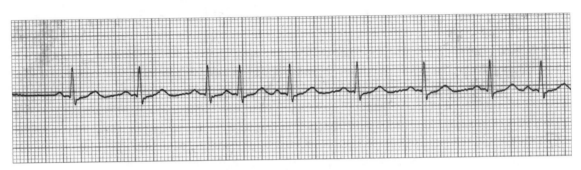

Sinus rhythm with a premature atrial complex.

❍ **What is a premature ventricular complex?**

It is a premature ventricular beat occurring earlier than the next expected ventricular beat.

❍ **What is a ventricular escape beat?**

Ventricular escape beats are beats which occur late in the cardiac cycle occurring after the next expected beat. Escape beats are protective in nature. Lidocaine should not be used to treat ventricular escape beats.

❍ **What is the following rhythm?**

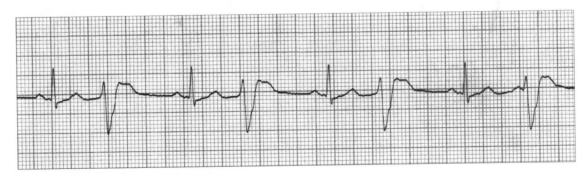

Sinus rhythm with ventricular bigeminy.

○   **What is the following rhythm?**

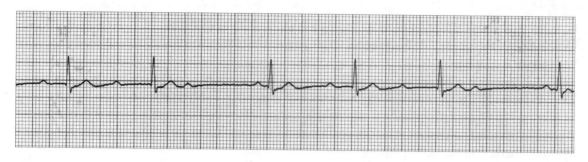

Second degree AV block, Mobitz Type I.

○   **What are the characteristics of second degree AV block, Mobitz Type I?**

- Rate: atrial rate is greater than ventricular rate
- Rhythm: atrial rhythm is regular, ventricular rhythm is irregular
- P waves: normal in size and configuration, T waves may not necessarily be followed by QRS
- P-R interval: lengthens with each cycle until a P wave appears without a QRS complex
- QRS: 0.10 seconds or less and is dropped periodically

○   **What is the following rhythm?**

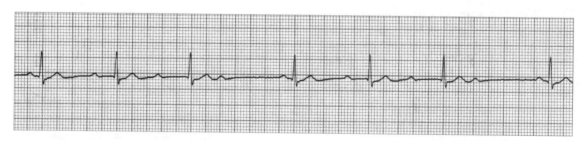

Second degree AV block, Mobitz Type I.

○   **What injuries are associated with electrocution?**

Cardiac effects include V-fib, asystole, and other serious dysrhythmias. In addition to cardiac effects, suspect closed head injury, peripheral nerve injury, myoglobinuria, and fractures.

○   **What is the most common forecaster of ischemic stroke?**

Transient ischemic attack.

❍ **Should the Heimlich maneuver be used on patients who have suffered near drowning?**

Typically no. The Heimlich maneuver is only used when a foreign body obstructing the airway is suspected.

❍ **What are the signs and symptoms of mild hypothermia?**

Cold, pale skin, decreased coordination, decreased judgment, memory loss, rise in blood pressure, and increased respiratory rate.

❍ **What are the signs and symptoms of moderate hypothermia?**

Decreased reflexes, no shivering, decreased respiratory rate, increased muscle rigidity, bradydysrhythmias, and decreased level of consciousness.

❍ **What are the signs and symptoms of severe hypothermia?**

Hypotension, stupor, rigidity, V-fib or asystole, undetectable pulse and respiratory rate.

❍ **Why is alternating current more dangerous than direct current?**

First, because the victim is frozen to the current and second, alternating current causes titanic muscle contractions.

❍ **T/F: Hand to hand accidental electric shock is the most dangerous form of electrocution.**

True. Hand to hand or the transthoracic pathway is the most likely to be fatal.

❍ **What is the prehospital treatment for a patient with cardiac arrest due to hypothermia?**

CPR, shock for V-fib or pulseless V-tach, intubate and ventilate, establish an IV and infuse saline. If a patient fails to respond to three defibrillation attempts as well as drug therapy, stop further shocks and transport to the hospital immediately.

❍ **What are the signs and symptoms of cocaine toxicity?**

Tachycardia, seizures, hypertension, dyspnea, agitation, confusion, hypothermia, respiratory depression, respiratory arrest, chest pain, and acute MI.

❍ **What is the primary concern in a near drowning victim?**

Management of hypoxemia.

○   **What factors impact electrical injuries?**

Amperage, voltage, pathway of current, type of current, resistance of tissues, and time of exposure.

○   **What is the recommended sequence of treatment for a loan rescuer with immediate access to a defibrillator?**

Access Responsiveness
Call for help
Open the airway
Confirm airway is unobstructed by giving 2 breaths
Confirm pulselessness
Defibrillate

○   **What are the signs and symptoms of a stroke?**

Weakness, change in vision, hearing loss, vertigo, nausea, vomiting, facial weakness, confusion, headache, and photophobia.

○   **In an acute cardiac arrest, what type of acidosis usually occurs?**

Respiratory and metabolic. Treat with increased ventilation. Sodium bicarbonate is not routinely given.

○   **What are the dangers associated with aspiration of gastric contents?**

Aspiration is potentially lethal. Aspiration may occur during CPR, following bag-valve-mask ventilation and with removal of an esophageal obturator airway.

○   **What is the primary treatment of acidosis during an acute cardiac arrest?**

Hyperventilation.

○   **A patient presents with sinus tachycardia, hyperventilation, and a blood pressure of 130/80. Auscultation reveals bibasilar rales. What therapy should be initiated?**

Pulmonary edema should be treated with oxygen, morphine, and furosemide.

○   **What is the most common dangerous rhythm following the onset of atraumatic cardiac arrest in adults?**

Ventricular fibrillation.

❍ **What is the most important step in the diagnosis of acute myocardial infarction?**

History.

❍ **A patient in the critical care unit complains of chest pressure. Blood pressure drops to 50/30 and the heart rate decreases to 30 beats per minute. What medication should be used first?**

Atropine (0.5-1 mg IVP). May be repeated if little or no response.

❍ **In a patient with an acute myocardial infarction what drug is most commonly used to relieve pain?**

Morphine.

❍ **After atropine, what is the next treatment for symptomatic bradycardia?**

External pacing, followed by transvenous pacing.

❍ **What are important effects of epinephrine?**

Increased peripheral vascular resistance and myocardial contractility. It may restore electrical activity in asystole and facilitate defibrillation in ventricular fibrillation.

❍ **What are complications of atropine?**

Tachycardia and ischemia.

❍ **What routes may nitroglycerin be administered?**

Sublingual, transdermal, or IV.

❍ **What is the most common side effect of nitroglycerin?**

Headache.

❍ **What is the most serious side effect of nitroglycerin?**

Hypotension.

❍ **T/F: Nitroglycerin may be harmful to patients on digitalis.**

False.

O   **What is the effect of low dose (1-2 mcg/kg/min) of dopamine?**

Renal vasodilatation.

O   **What is the primary adverse side effect of beta-blockers, such as propranolol, on the myocardium?**

Depression of myocardial contractility.

O   **What is the most common adverse reaction to bretylium?**

Hypotension.

O   **What are the potential side effects of isoproterenol?**

Arrhythmias and myocardial ischemia.

O   **What is the endpoint for the administration of procainamide?**

Hypotension, QRS widening more than 50% of pretreatment width, or a total of 17 mg/kg of the drug has been injected.

O   **What is the treatment for verapamil overdose?**

Calcium chloride.

O   **What drug is used to treat refractory ventricular fibrillation?**

Procainamide at 20mg/min IV infusion for a total dose of 17 mg/kg then continued infusion at 1-4 mg/min depending on success of treatment. Bretylium is no longer in use.

O   **T/F: Isoproterenol, a beta-adrenergic stimulant: increases myocardial irritability, heart rate, force of contraction, and may increase the size of a myocardial infarction.**

True.

O   **T/F: During cardiac arrest, sodium bicarbonate should be administered every five minutes to prevent metabolic acidosis.**

False.

O   **What are two common adverse reactions to bretylium IV?**

Vomiting and hypotension.

❍ **A patient presents with paroxysmal supraventricular tachycardia at a rate in excess of 250 beats per minute. The patient has not responded to vagal maneuvers. What is the next line of treatment?**

Adenosine 6 mg IVP. If no response, administer adenosine 12 mg IVP. If still no response, give another 12 mg IV push dose of adenosine.

❍ **T/F: In a hypothermic patient, endotracheal intubation should be withheld as it may precipitate cardiac arrest.**

False.

❍ **T/F: Hypothermic hearts are unresponsive to defibrillators or pacer stimuli.**

True.

❍ **T/F: Hypothermia reduces the effect of most drugs.**

True.

❍ **T/F: Core rewarming is indicated in the treatment of moderate hypothermia.**

True.

❍ **T/F: A patient has sustained a near drowning. The Heimlich maneuver should be used.**

False.

❍ **What is the most common arrhythmia seen after an AC current shock?**

Ventricular fibrillation.

❍ **A 36 year-old patient arrives to the emergency department with a history of palpitations. A rhythm strip demonstrates narrow-complex tachycardia with a rate of 240 beats per minute Blood pressure is 80/50. What should be the first intervention?**

Valsalva maneuver.

❍ **A 22 year-old patient with supraventricular tachycardia has been treated with a Valsalva maneuver and verapamil 5 mg IVP. The blood pressure suddenly falls to 50/palp and the heart rate climbs to 300 beats per minute. What is the next intervention?**

Synchronized cardioversion at 100 J.

○   **A 70 year-old patient presents to the emergency department with a history of recent myocardial infarction. On arrival, the patient is pulseless. The paramedics indicate that in the ambulance, the patient had ventricular tachycardia. What should be your first action?**

Countershock with 200 J of unsynchronized electricity.

○   **A 70 year-old presents with ventricular tachycardia. The patient is cool, clammy, and diaphoretic. Pulse is 150 beats per minute, blood pressure is 60/40, and the respiratory rate is 26. What is the initial treatment?**

Synchronized cardioversion at 100 J.

○   **T/F: Lidocaine is indicated in a patient with pulseless electrical activity.**

False. Treatment includes CPR, epinephrine, ventilation, and a rapid fluid challenge.

○   **A 60 year-old in the ICU complains of lightheadedness and weakness. Respiratory rate is 20. Blood pressure is 70/40. Pulse is 40 beats per minute. The monitor reveals the following rhythm. What would be the next treatment?**

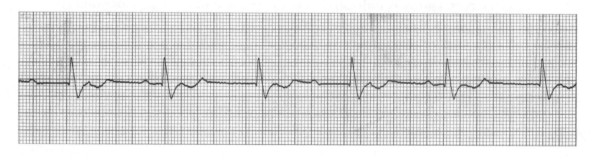

External pacemaker, followed by transvenous pacing.

○   **Treatment for a patient with acute ventricular fibrillation who is pulseless?**

Defibrillate at 200 J.

○   **A patient with known coronary artery disease presents with non-sustained ventricular tachycardia. The patient is hemodynamically stable. What is the treatment?**

Lidocaine 1-1.5 mg/kg IVP.

○   **You are performing synchronized cardioversion when ventricular fibrillation develops. What is your most immediate course of action?**

Countershock at 200 J unsynchronized.

○   A patient presents with CPR in progress. The patient has pulseless electrical activity. What is the first treatment to be given?

Epinephrine (1:10,000) 1 mg IVP.

○   An 80 year-old patient has the following rhythm. Blood pressure is 120/80. The patient is asymptomatic. The patient was previously treated with 3 mg/kg of lidocaine which has had no effect. What would be the next therapy?

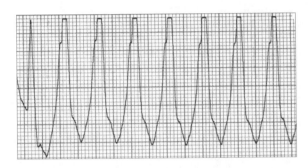

Discontinue lidocaine and start procainamide at 20 mg/min IV.

○   What are the conditions required to be found negligent in the delivery of healthcare to a patient?

Injury, and an act or omission must have been shown to have caused that injury.

○   T/F: An ACLS provider card certifies that a student has successfully completed the standards of the American Heart Association course.

False. The ACLS provider card demonstrates that a student has successfully completed an ACLS course according to the standards of the American Heart Association.

○   T/F: With CPR in progress, an automatic defibrillator can analyze the rhythm.

False.

○   T/F: Prior to attaching an automatic defibrillator, it is important to determine if there is a pulse.

True.

○   T/F: Do not touch the patient during the defibrillation phase of automatic defibrillation.

True.

○   **What is the following rhythm?**

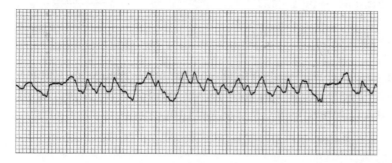

Ventricular fibrillation.

○   **What is the following rhythm?**

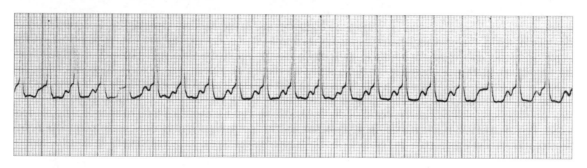

Atrial tachycardia.

○   **What is the following rhythm?**

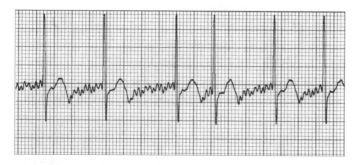

Atrial fibrillation.

○   **What is the following rhythm?**

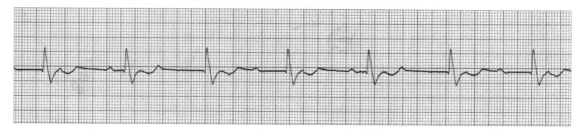

Third degree heart block.

○   **What is the following rhythm?**

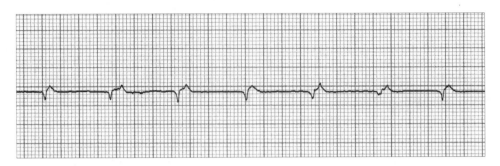

Accelerated junctional rhythm.

○   **What is the following rhythm?**

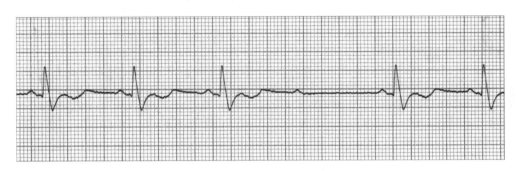

Second degree AV block, Mobitz Type II.

○   **What is the following rhythm?**

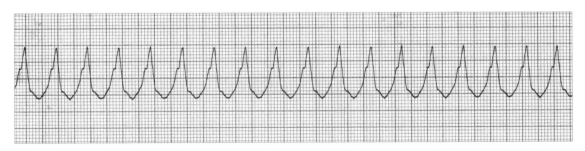

Ventricular tachycardia.

○   **T/F: Core rewarming is indicated in the treatment of moderate hypothermia.**

True.

○   **T/F: A patient has sustained a near drowning. The Heimlich maneuver should be used.**

False.

○   **What is the most common arrhythmia seen after an AC current shock?**

Ventricular fibrillation.

○   **A 36 year-old patient arrives to the emergency department with a history of palpitations. A rhythm strip demonstrates narrow-complex tachycardia with a rate of 240 beats per minute Blood pressure is 80/50. What should be the first intervention?**

Valsalva maneuver.

○   **A 22 year-old patient with supraventricular tachycardia has been treated with a Valsalva maneuver and verapamil 5 mg IVP. The blood pressure suddenly falls to 50/palp and the heart rate climbs to 300 beats per minute. What is the next intervention?**

Synchronized cardioversion at 100 J.

○   **A 70 year-old patient presents to the emergency department with a history of recent myocardial infarction. On arrival, the patient is pulseless. The paramedics indicate that in the ambulance, the patient had ventricular tachycardia. What should be your first action?**

Countershock with 200 J of unsynchronized electricity.

○   **A 70 year-old presents with ventricular tachycardia. The patient is cool, clammy, and diaphoretic. Pulse is 150 beats per minute, blood pressure is 60/40, and the respiratory rate is 26. What is the initial treatment?**

Synchronized cardioversion at 100 J.

○   **T/F: Lidocaine is indicated in a patient with pulseless electrical activity.**

False. Treatment includes CPR, epinephrine, ventilation, and a rapid fluid challenge.

○   **A 60 year-old in the ICU complains of lightheadedness and weakness. Respiratory rate is 20. Blood pressure is 70/40. Pulse is 40 beats per minute. The monitor reveals the following rhythm. What would be the next treatment?**

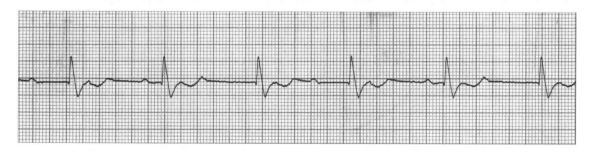

External pacemaker, followed by transvenous pacing.

○   **Treatment for a patient with acute ventricular fibrillation who is pulseless?**

Defibrillate at 200 J.

○   **A patient with known coronary artery disease presents with non-sustained ventricular tachycardia.   The patient is hemodynamically stable.   What is the treatment?**

Lidocaine 1-1.5 mg/kg IVP.

○   **You are performing synchronized cardioversion when ventricular fibrillation develops. What is your most immediate course of action?**

Countershock at 200 J unsynchronized.

○   **A patient presents with CPR in progress.   The patient has pulseless electrical activity. What is the first treatment to be given?**

Epinephrine (1:10,000) 1 mg IVP. If no IV access has been obtained, epinephrine can be given down the endotracheal tube (ETT) at 2.0 to 2.5 mg diluted in 10 ml of normal saline (2.0-2.5 ml of 1:1,000).

○   **An 80 year-old patient has the following rhythm.   Blood pressure is 120/80. The patient is asymptomatic.   The patient was previously treated with 3 mg/kg of lidocaine which has had no effect.   What would be the next therapy?**

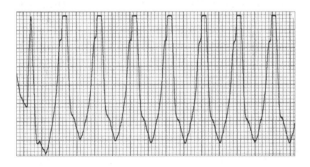

The rhythm strip shows monomorphic ventricular tachycardia.   Since the patient is hemodynamically stable at the present time, the next most appropriate therapy is amiodarone 150 mg IVP over 10 minutes, if the patient's ejection fraction is poor. If the patient's ejection fraction is well preserved, then procainamide at 20 mg/minute IV infusion up to a loading dose of 17 mg/kg, Amiodarone 150 mg IVP over 10 minutes, or Sotalol 160-320 mg po now and every 12 hours would be appropriate. Synchronized cardioversion starting at 100 joules should be immediately performed if the patient becomes hemodynamically unstable or pulseless at any point, if the above modalities for monomorphic stable VT fail, or if provider is not comfortable with the arrhythmia or clinical status of the patient.   For polymorphic stable ventricular tachycardia with prolonged QT interval, correction of electrolyte disorders (hyperkalemia, hypocalcemia) should be done promptly, and magnesium sulfate 1-2 grams IV, overdrive pacing, dilantin, or synchronized cardioversion at 100 J should be administered. For polymorphic VT with normal QT interval, beta-blockers, amiodarone, procainamide, sotalol or synchronized cardioversion can be administered.

○   **What are the conditions required to be found negligent in the delivery of healthcare to a patient?**

Injury, and an act or omission must have been shown to have caused that injury.

○   **T/F: An ACLS provider card certifies that a student has successfully completed the standards of the American Heart Association course.**

True. The ACLS provider card certifies that a student has successfully completed an ACLS course according to the standards of the American Heart Association.

○   **T/F: With CPR in progress, an automatic defibrillator can analyze the rhythm.**

False. The only rhythms that an automatic external defibrillator (AED) can analyze are ventricular tachycardia and ventricular fibrillation.

○   **T/F: Prior to attaching an automatic defibrillator, it is important to determine if there is a pulse.**

True.

○   **T/F: Do not touch the patient during the defibrillation phase of automatic defibrillation.**

True.

○   **What is the following rhythm?**

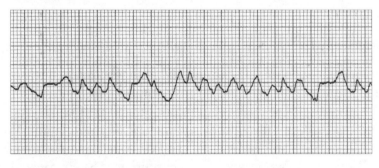

Ventricular fibrillation.

○ **What is the following rhythm?**

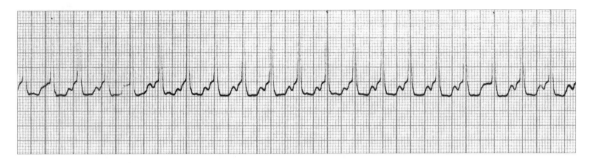

Atrial tachycardia.

○ **What is the following rhythm?**

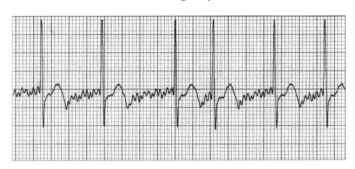

Atrial fibrillation.

○ **What is the following rhythm?**

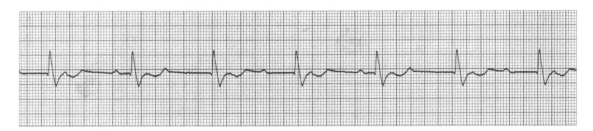

Third degree heart block.

○ **What is the following rhythm?**

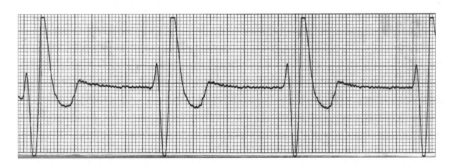

Idioventricular rhythm.

○   **What is the following rhythm?**

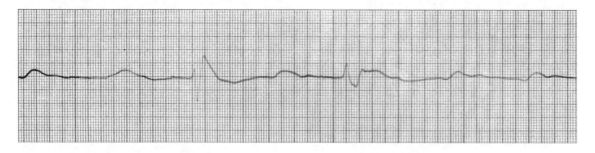

Agonal rhythm.

○   **What is the following rhythm?**

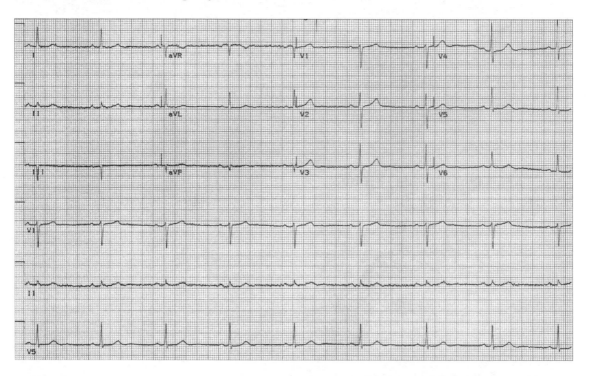

Sinus bradycardia.

○   **What is the following rhythm?**

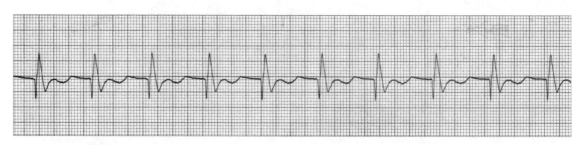

Ventricular paced rhythm.

○   **What is the following rhythm?**

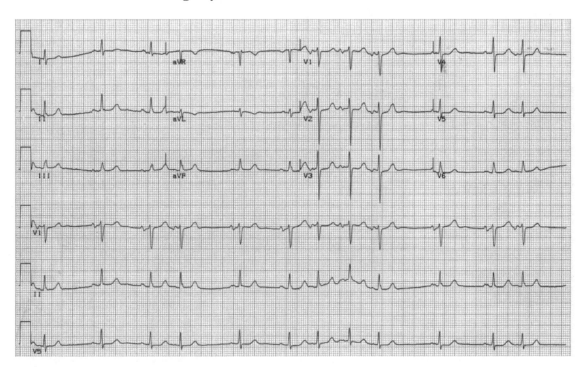

Sinus rhythm with frequent PACs.

○   **What is the following rhythm?**

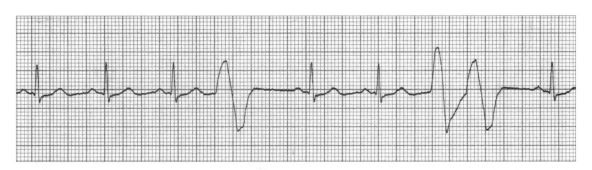

Sinus rhythm with frequent multifocal PVCs.

○   **What is the following rhythm?**

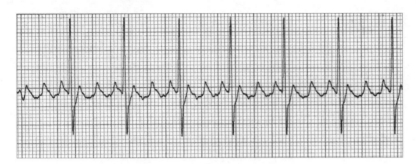

Atrial flutter.

○   **What is the following rhythm?**

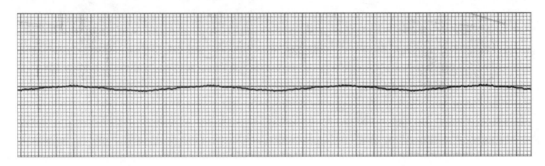

Asystole.

○   **What is the following rhythm?**

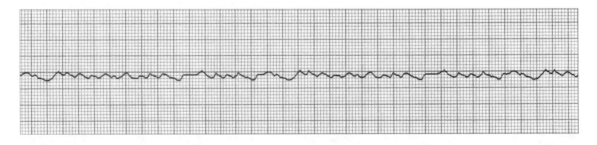

Ventricular fibrillation.

❍　**A patient presents with apnea and, is pulseless and unresponsive. The rhythm is as follows. What is the treatment?**

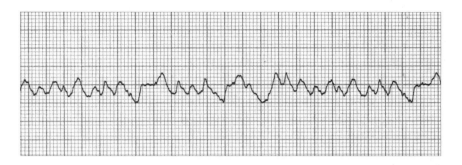

Immediately defibrillate with 200J, then 300J, and then 360 J; intubate the patient, and obtain IV access.

❍　**A patient presents pulseless and unresponsive with the following strip. CPR and bag-mask ventilation is in progress and IV access has been obtained. What is the condition and what is the treatment?**

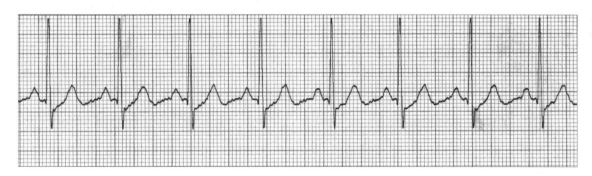

Pulseless electrical activity. Continue CPR, intubate and give epinephrine 1 mg IVP now and every 3-5 minutes. (The rhythm strip, although it looks like sinus rhythm is pulseless electrical activity in a pulseless, unresponsive patient).

❍　**T/F: Endotracheal intubation reduces the risk of aspiration of gastric contents.**

True.

❍　**T/F: Sodium bicarbonate may be added to an IV containing catecholamines.**

False.

❍　**T/F: Sodium bicarbonate is recommended early in cardiac arrest management.**

False.

❍   T/F: Epinephrine increases peripheral vascular resistance and increases myocardial contractility.

True.

❍   T/F: Atropine is used to treat ventricular tachycardia.

False.

❍   What effect does isoproterenol have on the heart?

It increases heart rate, force of contraction, and myocardial irritability.

❍   A 70 year-old presents with chest pain with radiation into the arm. The chest pain has lasted a period of 90 minutes. No relief was obtained with nitroglycerin. Blood pressure is 120/80 and pulse is 110. ECG shows no evidence of myocardial infarction. What drug should be administered?

The patient should be treated with morphine 2-10 mg IV to relieve pain.

❍   What is the most common cause of sudden death?

Ventricular fibrillation.

❍   T/F: After a stressful incident, health care worker debriefing should occur.

True.

❍   What is the treatment for a patient with hemorrhagic or hypovolemic shock?

Rapid fluid infusion.

❍   In an adult, after two unsuccessful defibrillation attempts, what energy should be used for the third attempt?

360 J.

❍   A patient with pulseless electrical activity is undergoing CPR. Exam reveals distended neck veins. What diagnosis should be considered and how should it be ruled out?

Cardiac tamponade should be ruled out by performing pericardiocentesis.

❍   **In a patient with serious signs and symptoms, what is the treatment for ventricular tachycardia?**

Synchronized cardioversion.

❍   **What is the treatment for a 40 year-old patient whose blood pressure is 60/30 mmHg and has the following rhythm seen below?**

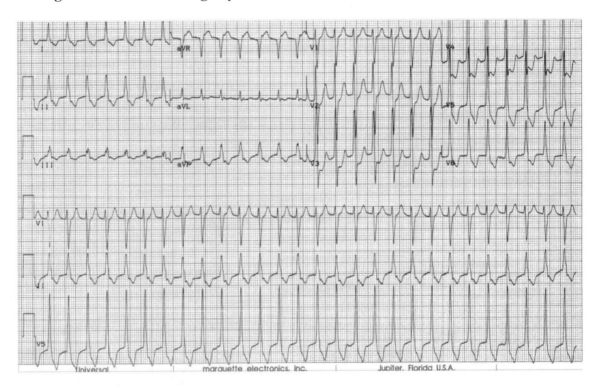

Synchronized cardioversion with 50-100J.   (The ECG above shows supraventricular tachycardia).

❍   **What is the most common cause of pulseless electrical activity?**

Hypovolemia. Other causes include tension pneumothorax and pericardial tamponade.

❍   **When is it medically and legally acceptable to terminate CPR?**

When the cardiovascular system has failed to respond to reasonable BLS and ACLS efforts.

❍   **In adult defibrillation, how many pounds of pressure should be placed on each electric paddle?**

Twenty-five.

O   **A patient with ventricular fibrillation has been resuscitated using no antiarrhythmic drugs. Once the pulse is restored, what drugs should be provided?**

Oxygen and intravenous lidocaine.

O   **T/F: A poor result after resuscitation is evidence of negligence.**

False.

O   **What is the first drug used to treat a patient with pulseless electrical activity.**

Epinephrine, 1 mg/kg IVP now and every 3-5 minutes for the duration of ACLS protocol.

O   **An overdose patient is unresponsive with spontaneous respirations. In what position should they be placed?**

Recovery position.

O   **What is the effect of a dopamine infusion at greater than 5 mcg/kg/minute?**

Peripheral artery vasoconstriction.

O   **What are common risk factors for coronary artery disease?**

Family history of coronary artery disease, hypertension, diabetes mellitus, hyperlipidemia and tobacco use.

O   **In a cardiac arrest patient without an IV, how should epinephrine and atropine be administered?**

Down the endotracheal tube.

O   **How is isoproterenol dosed?**

Dosage is 2-10 mcg/minute IV drip titrated to response.

O   **Why should leg veins be avoided for IV therapy?**

High deep venous thrombosis risk.

O   **How should CPR be performed in a pregnant patient with acute cardiac arrest?**

Left lateral position to move the uterus off the vena cava during CPR.

❍ **Name five causes of pulseless electrical activity.**

Cardiac tamponade, tension pneumothorax, hypovolemia, myocardial rupture, and massive pulmonary embolism. Also hypoxia, acidosis, and drug overdose can cause pulseless electrical activity.

❍ **T/F: Ventricular fibrillation produces no cardiac output.**

True.

❍ **T/F: A potential complication of transcutaneous pacing is injury to the operator by electric shock.**

False.

❍ **A patient is apneic and pulseless. The following is the presenting rhythm. Treatment?**

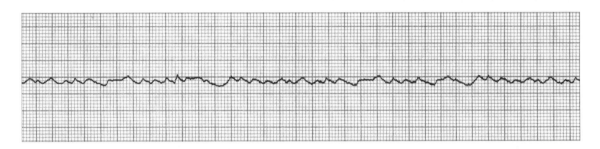

Defibrillate with 200J, 200-300J, then 360J. If no response, inubate and ventilate patient for immediate oxygen delivery, and obtain IV access as soon as possible. (The rhythm shown is ventricular fibrillation). Administer Epinephrine 1 mg IVP (or 2 mg down the ETT), or Vasopressin 40 units IVP (one time dose) and repeat the defibrillation and algorhythm sequence in 1-2 minutes if no response.

❍ **The patient is pulseless and apneic with the following rhythm. Bag-mask ventilations and chest compressions are begun. What should be the initial treatment?**

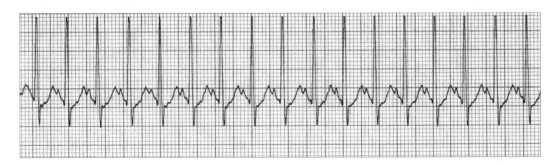

CPR, intubate, administer epinephrine IV. (The above rhythm is pulseless electrical activity).

○   **A patient complains of chest pain. BP is 150/80. Respirations are 24/min. The rhythm is as follows below. What should be the initial treatment?**

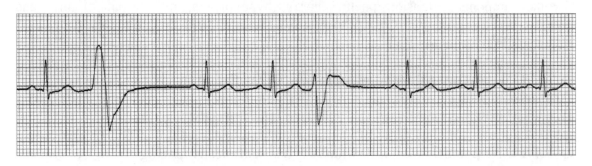

O2, IV access, nitroglycerin, morphine, and lidocaine. (The rhythm above shows normal sinus rhythm with polymorphic PVC's).

○   **A patient complains of nausea, weakness, and shortness of breath. The patient is cool and clammy. BP 70/50, pulse 30, respirations 28. The monitor shows the following rhythm. What should be the order of treatment?**

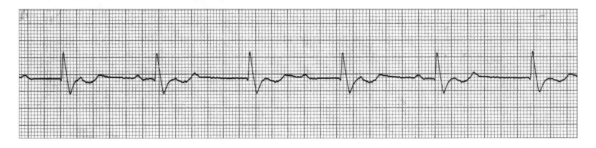

O2, atropine, pacemaker, dopamine, epinephrine, isoproterenol. (The rhythm above shows 3° AV block).

○   **An 80 year-old complains of chest pain which began one hour ago. The patient is pale and diaphoretic. BP is 80/50, respiratory rate is 24. The monitor shows the following rhythm. What should be the initial treatment?**

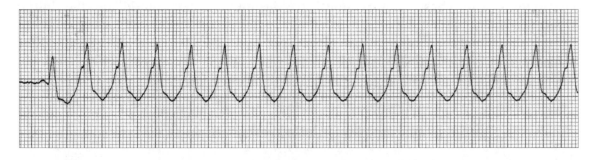

Consider sedation and synchronized countershock with 100J. (The rhythm shows ventricular tachycardia).

○   **You are called to the room of an awake patient complaining of nausea, chest pain and dizziness. The patient is cool to the touch. Exam reveals a BP of 70/40 and a respiratory rate of 22/min. The monitor shows the following rhythm. What should be the initial treatment?**

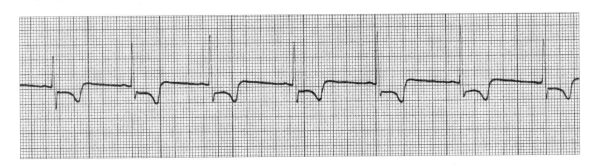

O2, IV access, intravenous atropine, fluid bolus and/or dopamine infusion. (The rhythm above shows sinus bradycardia with ischemic-type ST depression and T inversion).

○   **A patient in the CCU complains of sudden dizziness, nausea, vomiting, and difficulty breathing. Exam reveals rales throughout both lung fields, BP is 80/50, and respirations are 40/min. The monitor shows the following rhythm. What should be the initial treatment?**

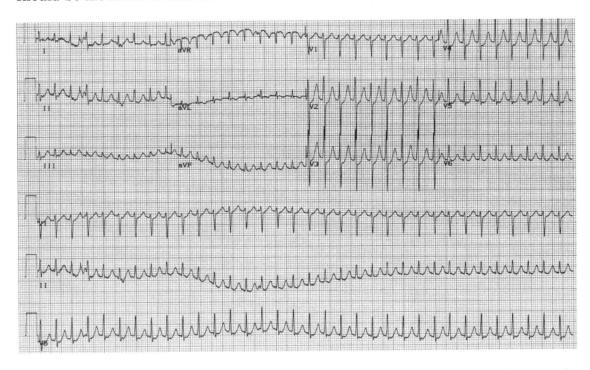

IV access, O2, monitor. Give IV sedation, then perform synchronized cardioversion at 100J. (The ECG above shows paroxysmal supraventricular tachycardia).

○   **The patient has been in the following rhythm for 2 - 3 minutes. What should be the initial treatment?**

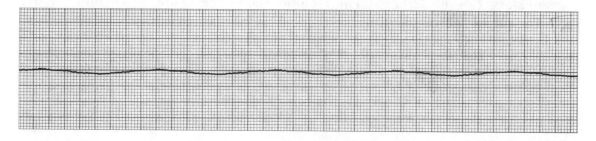

CPR, epinephrine, atropine. May consider transvenous pacemaker. (The rhythm above shows asystole).

○   **A patient is pulseless and apneic. CPR is in progress. The monitor shows the following rhythm. What should be the initial treatment?**

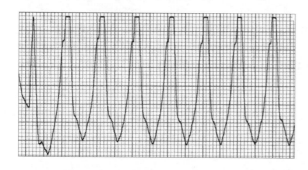

Defibrillate immediately with 200J, 200-300J, 360J, intubate, IV access. (The rhythm above shows ventricular tachycardia).

○   **The patient "fainted". Exam reveals an alert patient. BP is 120/80 and respirations are 16/min. The patient denies chest pain or injuries. The monitor shows the following rhythm. What should be the treatment?**

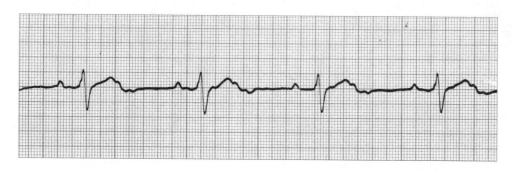

O2, IV access, transcutaneous pacemaker on standby, monitor closely and rapid transport to a facility for likely permanent pacemaker implantation. (The rhythm above shows 2° AV block, Mobitz Type II).

O   **What is the most important goal of ACLS?**

Cerebral resuscitation.

O   **What is the single most important ACLS intervention?**

Identification and treatment of ventricular fibrillation.

O   **What is the differential diagnosis of a flat line on the rhythm strip?**

Loose leads, leads not connected, monitor not connected, no power, signal gain too low, isoelectric VF/VT, and true asystole.

O   **When is a precordial thump used?**

In a witnessed arrest, when no pulse is present and no defibrillator is immediately available.

O   **What is the treatment sequence for VF/VT?**

Defibrillate, protect the airway, and ventilate the patient.

O   **T/F: Defibrillation "jump starts" the heart?**

False. Defibrillation actually produces temporary asystole.

O   **Should the pulse be checked between shocks in a patient that displays persistent VF/VT?**

Yes. The pulse and rhythm should be checked after all defibrillations.

O   **Can a nitroglycerin patch explode during defibrillation?**

No, but they can cause smoke, explosive noises, visible arcing, and burns and, thus, should be removed prior to defibrillation.

O   **What precautions should be taken when defibrillating a patient with an implanted pacemaker or automatic cardiovertor-defibrillator?**

Avoid placing defibrillator pads over the generator unit or device. Defibrillation over the unit may block part of the defibrillation current or disable the implanted device.

O   **In a patient with a hypothermic cardiac arrest that remains in VF/VT after three defibrillations, what should be done next if VF/VT persists?**

Intubate and obtain IV access.

O   **What is the treatment algorithm for persistent VF/Pulseless VT?**

Primary ABCD survey (check responsiveness, activate emergency response system, call for defibrillator, open the airway, provide positive pressure ventilations) > CPR > Check for VF/VT on defibrillator, Defibrillate up to three times at 200 J, 200-300J, 360 J (or equivalent biphasic) (checking pulse and rhythm after each defibrillation) > Secondary ABCD survey (Continue CPR) > Intubate and establish IV > Epinephrine 1 mg IVP q 3-5 min or Vasopressin 40 units IVP (one time dose) > Defibrillate within 30-60s > Lidocaine 1.0 mg-1.5 mg/kg IVP q 3-5 min max 3 mg/kg or Amiodarone 300 mg IVP > Magnesium sulfate 1-2 g IV in Torsades de Pointes or suspected hypomagnesemic state refractory to VF > Procainamide 20 mg/min to max of 17 mg/kg > Sodium Bicarbonate 1 mEq/kg IV if known acidosis, tricyclic overdose, long arrest (>10 minutes), and in hypoxic lactic acidosis > Defibrillate at 360 J (or equivalent biphasic), 30-60 s after each dose of medication (drug-shock, drug-shock, etc.).

O   **What are the indications for sodium bicarbonate in an acute cardiac arrest?**

Known acidosis, hyperkalemia, tricyclic overdose, long arrest (>10 minutes), and in hypoxic lactic acidosis.

O   **What effect does epinephrine have on blood flow to the brain and heart?**

Increases blood flow to both the heart and brain.

O   **What is the differential diagnosis of pulseless electrical activity?**

Hypovolemia, hypoxia, cardiac tamponade, tension pneumothorax, hypothermia, massive pulmonary embolism, drug overdose, hyperkalemia, preexisting acidosis, and massive MI.

O   **What is the treatment for hyperkalemia?**

First treatment should be intravenous Calcium chloride, followed by intravenous Regular insulin, glucose, sodium bicarbonate, and sodium polystyrene sulfonate/sorbitol (Kayexalate) every 4-6 hours until normalization of the serum potassium level is achieved. If this fails to normalize the potassium level, hemodialysis should be employed.

O   **What is pulseless electrical activity?**

Absence of a pulse in the presence of some type of electrical activity, other than ventricular fibrillation.

○   **What is the most common cause of electrical activity without measurable blood pressure?**

Hypovolemia. Diagnose by history and look for flat neck veins.

○   **What is the treatment algorithm for Pulseless Electrical Activity?**

CPR > Intubate and establish IV > Check blood flow > Consider causes: Hypovolemia (volume infusion), Hypoxia (ventilate), Cardiac tamponade (pericardiocentesis), Tension pneumothorax (needle decompression), Hypothermia (rewarming), Massive pulmonary embolism (surgery, thrombolytics), Drug overdose (charcoal, lavage), Hyperkalemia (calcium chloride, insulin, glucose, bicarb, sodium polystyrene, dialysis), Acidosis (bicarb), Massive MI (thrombolytics, PTCA) > Epinephrine 1 mg IVP q 3-5 min > if rhythm shows bradycardia, give atropine 1 mg IVP q 3-5 min to total of 0.03-0.04 mg/kg.

○   **How can you confirm asystole on the monitor?**

Change to another lead on the lead-select switch or change placement of the defibrillation paddles by 90 degrees.

○   **What is the asystole treatment algorithm?**

CPR > Intubate and establish IV > Confirm asystole in 2 leads > Consider causes: hypoxia, hyperkalemia, hypokalemia, preexisting acidosis, drug overdose, and hypothermia > Epinephrine 1 mg IVP q 3-5 min > Atropine 1 mg IVP q 3-5 min up to 0.03-0.04 mg/kg > consider immediate transcutaneous pacing.

○   **How should post-resuscitation arrhythmias be treated?**

As a general rule, most should be left untreated for the immediate post-resuscitation period.

○   **What is the bradycardia treatment algorithm?**

ABCs > establish IV, O2, Monitor > H & P > 12-lead ECG > CXR >Serious symptoms > Atropine 0.5-1.0 mg IV push > Transcutaneous pacer > Dopamine 5-20 mcg/kg/min > Epinephrine 2-10 mcg/min > isoproterenol.

○   **Should lidocaine be used to treat third-degree heart block with ventricular escape beats?**

No, it could in fact be lethal. Lidocaine suppresses ventricular escape depolarizations and could suppress the wide-complex QRS ventricular escape beats that are found in complete heart block, thus resulting in asystole.

○ **What is the effect of dopamine at low-doses (1-4 mcg/kg/minute)?**

Renal dose: Dopaminergic effect that causes mesenteric, renal, and cerebral vascular dilation. Used to treat low renal output.

○ **What is the effect of dopamine at intermediate doses (5-10 mcg/kg/minute)?**

Cardiac dose: Beta-1 and alpha-adrenergic effect causing enhanced myocardial contractility, increased cardiac output, and a rise in blood pressure. Used to treat symptomatic bradycardias.

○ **What is the effect of dopamine at high doses (10-20 mcg/kg/minute)?**

Vasopressor dose: Alpha-adrenergic effect causing peripheral arterial and venous vasoconstriction. Used to treat low blood pressure and shock.

○ **What is the treatment algorithm for stable atrial fibrillation and atrial flutter?**

ABCs > O2, establish IV, Monitor, Vital signs > H & P > Obtain 12-lead ECG > PCXR > Consider Diltiazem, Beta-blockers, verapamil, Digoxin, Procainamide > Quinidine > intravenous Ibutilide. Anticoagulants are strongly recommended when acuity of onset of atrial fibrillation is unknown.

○ **What is the treatment algorithm for stable paroxysmal supraventricular tachycardia?**

ABCs > O2, establish IV, Monitor, Vital signs > brief H & P > Obtain 12-lead ECG > PCXR > Vagal maneuvers > Adenosine 6 mg IVP over 1-3 s repeated in 1-2 min at a dose of 12 mg rapid IVP repeated at 12 to 18 mg > verapamil 5 mg IV, then 5-10 mg IV > Consider Digoxin, intravenous beta- blockers, and intravenous Diltiazem.

○ **What is the treatment algorithm for stable wide-complex QRS tachycardia?**

ABCs > O2, establish IV, Monitor, Vital signs > brief H & P > Obtain 12-lead ECG > order portable CXR > Lidocaine 1-1.5 mg/kg IVP q 5-10 min repeat at 0.50-0.75 mg/kg IVP, max total 3 mg/kg > Procainamide 20 mg/min, max 17 mg/kg > Synchronized cardioversion at 100 joules.

○ **What is the treatment algorithm for unstable wide-complex QRS tachycardia (rate > 150)?**

ABCs > O2, establish IV, Monitor, Vital signs > Order 12-lead ECG > Order portable CXR > Immediate unsynchronized cardioversion 200 J, 200-300 J, 360 J (check pulse and rhythm after each cardioversion attempt) > Alternate Drug – Shock, Drug – Shock --- Lidocaine 1-1.5 mg/kg IVP q 5-10 min repeat at 0.50-0.75 mg/kg IVP, max total 3 mg/kg > Procainamide 20 mg/min, max 17 mg/kg.

❍ **Discontinuing patient care before transferring care to another healthcare provider with equal or greater training is called _____.**

Abandonment.

❍ **The obligation to provide care is a concept known as _____.**

Duty to act.

❍ **A systolic blood pressure of < 90, weak rapid pulse, and diaphoresis are signs of what?**

Shock.

❍ **Congestive heart failure usually starts with failure in which portion of the heart?**

Left ventricle.

❍ **When preparing to insert an oropharyngeal airway, what other equipment should you have available to you?**

Suction, bag-valve mask, and oxygen.

❍ **Two differences between heat stroke and heat exhaustion are?**

Heat stroke presents with dry hot skin and rapid pulse; heat exhaustion presents with heavy perspiration and a weak pulse.

❍ **What is a normal systolic blood pressure for an adult?**

100 plus the age up to 140 mmHg, 10 less for females.

❍ **How do you measure blood pressure by palpation?**

Pump up the cuff until you lose the radial pulse + 20 mmHg, then release the air until the radial pulse returns.

❍ **What artery is compressed when you take a blood pressure on the upper arm?**

The brachial artery.

❍ **What is the minimum systolic blood pressure if you can feel a radial pulse?**

80.

❍ **Name the artery used to check circulation on an adult during the primary assessment.**

The carotid artery.

❍ **Small airways throughout the respiratory system are easily blocked by _____.**

Secretions and swelling of the airway.

❍ **What is the purpose of examining a child from the trunk to head approach?**

This is done to build confidence and to help relieve anxiety in the ill or injured child.

❍ **General impression of a well as opposed to a sick child can be obtained from inspection of overall appearance. List three signs you use to obtain a generalized impression of the patient.**

Mental status, effort of breathing, skin color.

❍ **T/F: It is proper treatment to provide oxygen and assist ventilation in a child with cyanosis and poor muscle tone.**

True.

❍ **Describe the signs and symptoms of a child in shock.**

Rapid respiratory rate, pale cool clammy skin, weak or absent peripheral pulses and delayed capillary refill.

❍ **After the child is removed from the water, what is the top priority in near drowning cases?**

Artificial ventilation.

❍ **What is the single most important maneuver to ensure an open airway in a child with a suspected head and neck injury?**

The modified jaw thrust.

○ **What procedure should be used to open an airway in an unconscious child?**

Jaw thrust.

○ **Why should you avoid letting air into the stomach when ventilating a patient?**

Air in the stomach can distend the abdomen and interfere with artificial ventilation efforts.

○ **What complications can arise from a tracheostomy tube?**

Displacement, obstruction, bleeding, infection and air leakage.

○ **Describe the three steps of alveolar capillary exchange.**

Oxygen-rich air enters the alveoli during each respiration.
Oxygen-poor blood in the capillaries passes into the alveoli.
Oxygen enters the capillaries as carbon dioxide enters the alveoli.

○ **Describe the two steps of capillary/cellular exchange.**

Cells give up carbon dioxide to the capillaries.
Capillaries give up oxygen to the cells.

AIRWAY MANAGEMENT

❍ **What are the complications of a cricothyroidotomy?**

Esophageal or tracheal laceration, hemorrhage, hematoma formation, aspiration, hoarseness, asphyxia, vocal cord paralysis, mediastinal emphysema, and creation of a false passage.

❍ **What are the advantages of the pharyngotracheal lumen airway?**

Eliminates the need for an air mask, airway visualization is not required, and avoids hyperextension of the neck.

❍ **Why is cricoid pressure applied?**

Assists in placement of the endotracheal tube and minimizes gastric aspiration.

❍ **When using a face mask, what is the minimum oxygen flow rate that can be used?**

5 L/min. Lower rates lead to accumulation of inhaled air in the reservoir.

❍ **What is the maximum length of time that a patient should be suctioned?**

10 seconds.

❍ **What is the maximum length of time that should be spent on an intubation attempt?**

30 seconds, by American Heart Association guidelines.

❍ **Where should the incision be made in performing a cricothyroidotomy?**

Incise the cricothyroid membrane. The superior landmark is the notch at the base of the thyroid cartilage and the inferior landmark is the cricoid cartilage.

❍ **Why avoid a pop-off valve on a bag-valve device during an acute respiratory arrest?**

High airway pressures may be needed to ventilate the lungs and a pop-off valve may prevent delivery of sufficient tidal volume.

❍   **What are the signs and symptoms of respiratory distress?**

Dyspnea, retractions, nasal flaring, tracheal tugging, jugular venous distention, difficulty speaking, and confusion.

❍   **What are the indications for needle cricothyroidotomy?**

Upper airway obstruction that cannot be relieved by oral or nasal intubation.

❍   **T/F: Cricothyroidotomy is used in patients with severe edema of the glottis, oral and facial injuries, oral hemorrhage, and in the presents of laryngeal fractures.**

True.

❍   **What are contraindications to the esophageal airway?**

Avoid in conscious patients, children under the age of 16, esophageal disease such as cancer and caustic substance ingestion. The EOA should be removed within two hours.

❍   **When intubating a patient, how far should the endotracheal tube cuff be advanced past the vocal cords?**

1 to 2.5 cm.

❍   **T/F: The oropharyngeal airway prevents biting of the endotracheal tube, allows suctioning, and prevents airway obstruction.**

True.

❍   **What are the contraindications of the pharyngotracheal lumen airway?**

Patients less than 14 years of age, caustic ingestions, semiconscious patients with a gag reflex, and esophageal disease or injury.

❍   **What are the indications for endotracheal intubation?**

Lack of gag reflex, inability to protect the airway, difficulty ventilating the patient, and cardiac arrest with ongoing chest compressions.

❍   **An 8 year-old is found by paramedics to be short of breath. What should be used to provide supplemental oxygen to a conscious child?**

Oxygen mask or nasal cannula.

❍   **In an infant, what are the signs and symptoms of acute respiratory failure?**

Increased respiratory rate, increased respiratory effort, poor skeletal muscle tone, retractions, cyanosis, and decreased level of consciousness.

❍   **In infants and children, what is the most common problem leading to cardiopulmonary arrest?**

Respiratory.

❍   **What are the advantages of endotracheal intubation?**

Protects the airway, reduces the risk of gastric distention, and provides a route for drug administration.

❍   **How long can endotracheal suction can be applied?**

Less than 10 seconds.

❍   **What is the most common problem with bag-valve-mask device use?**

Getting an adequate seal around the mouth and nose.

❍   **Endotracheal intubation is most appropriate in what type of patient?**

Comatose without a gag reflex.

❍   **Can pressure-cycled, oxygen-powered mechanical devices be used during CPR?**

No. Use manually triggered mechanical breathing devices.

❍   **What type of airway is the best choice for an unconscious patient with no gag reflex?**

Endotracheal intubation.

❍   **Following intubation, what is the most common cause of decreased or absent breath sounds?**

Endotracheal tube inserted into the right main stem bronchus.

❍   **A patient is intubated. Breath sounds cannot be auscultated. What is the most likely cause?**

Esophageal intubation.

❍ **What is the concern with using an oropharyngeal airway in a semiconscious patient?**

Vomiting or laryngospasm.

❍ **T/F: Esophageal obturator airways are contraindicated in children.**

True.

❍ **T/F: Bag-valve-mask devices provide close to 100% oxygen if a high flow rate is used and a reservoir is attached.**

True. The flow rate must be at 15 liters per minute.

❍ **Normal resting breathing rate for adults is _____ to _____ per minute.**

12 to 20.

❍ **A radial pulse should be assessed in patients 12 months or older. In patients less than 12 months, a _____ pulse should be assessed.**

Brachial.

❍ **The oxygen liter flow for a nasal cannula ranges between _____ and _____ liters per minute (lpm).**

2 and 6.

❍ **The oxygen liter flow for a medium flow (simple) mask ranges between _____ and _____ lpm.**

6 and 10.

❍ **The oxygen liter flow for a non-rebreather mask should be at least _____ lpm.**

15.

❍ **If a spinal injury is suspected, the _____ is used to bring the patient's head and neck in a neutral position.**

Jaw thrust maneuver.

❍ **Normal resting heart rate for an adult is _____ to _____ beats per minute.**

60 to 80.

○   To assess breathing, use the _____, _____ and _____ method.

Look, listen and feel.

○   When assessing respirations, it is necessary to note _____, _____ and _____.

Rate, quality and depth.

○   You arrive on scene of a 61 year-old male patient clutching his chest, complaining of chest pain, and in respiratory distress. What method of oxygen delivery would you use?

Non-rebreather mask.

○   The tongue is large relative to the small mandible and can block the airway in _____.

An unconscious child or infant.

○   Describe how the positioning of the airway is different in infants and children than in adults.

Do not hyperextend the neck.

○   Explain why suctioning a secretion-filled nasopharynx can improve breathing in an infant.

Infants are obligate nose breathers; therefore, suctioning can improve breathing.

○   Describe two ways children with dyspnea can compensate for short periods of time.

Children compensate by increasing their breathing rate, and increasing the effort of breathing.

○   Describe the technique used to open the airway in an infant or child.

Head-tilt, chin-lift; do not hyperextend.

○   What technique is used in opening a pediatric airway with suspected spinal injury?

Jaw thrust.

○   **Describe the procedure for clearing a complete airway obstruction in infants less that 1 year-old.**

Five back blows / 5 chest thrusts followed by foreign body removal only if you can see the foreign body. If the foreign body is not visible, then provide two breaths.

○   **Describe the procedure for clearing a complete airway obstruction in children greater than 1 year old.**

Five abdominal thrusts and foreign body removal only if visible.

○   **T/F: Toddlers will easily tolerate wearing an oxygen mask.**

False.

○   **Describe the three steps of inserting an oropharyngeal airway using a tongue blade.**

Insert tongue blade to the base of the tongue. Push down against the tongue while lifting upward. Insert oropharyngeal airway directly without rotation.

○   **Describe the proper technique for using a bag-valve-mask.**

Hold the mask down over the nose and seal around the mouth and mandible with the left hand. Make sure there are no air leaks. Squeeze bag slowly and evenly enough to make sure the chest rises adequately.

○   **What is the proper ventilatory rate for children and infants?**

One breath every 3 seconds or 20 breaths per minute.

○   **How can you assess if you are properly using the bag-valve-mask device?**

Breath sounds should be heard in the lungs bilaterally and visualization of the chest rising bilaterally.

○   **Seven items can be assessed to determine respiratory status in a pediatric patient. What are they?**

Note chest expansion/symmetry; effort of breathing; nasal flaring; retractions; grunting; respiratory rate/quality; stridor, crowing or noisy respirations.

○   **Stridor, crowing or noisy respirations are all signs of what type of respiratory distress?**

Partial airway obstruction.

○ **T/F: Children with a partial airway obstruction should be removed from their parents and placed in a supine position.**

False. Children should be assisted to the sitting position and can remain with the parents.

○ **Describe how you can deliver oxygen to a child who will not tolerate a nasal cannula or facemask.**

Hold tubing two inches from the child's face or place the tubing into the bottom of a paper cup and hold it near the child's face.

○ **Complete airway obstruction is an extreme emergency. You must be able to recognize the signs of complete airway obstruction. What are they?**

No crying noise, no coughing noise, inability to speak, cyanosis.

○ **A pediatric patient is said to be in respiratory arrest if his or her respiratory rate is less than _____ per minute.**

10.

○ **When should oxygen be given to a child in respiratory distress?**

Always.

○ **The proper treatment for a child in respiratory distress and altered mental status will include the following:**

Provide oxygen and assist ventilation with a bag-valve–mask.

○ **What is the emergency medical care for a child with complications associated with the tracheostomy tube?**

Maintain an open airway, ventilate and suction as needed, maintain a position of comfort and transport.

○ **You are adequately ventilating a patient when _____, _____, and _____.**

The chest rises and falls with each ventilation, the rate is appropriate to the age, and the heart rate returns to normal.

○ **Artificial ventilation is inadequate when _____, _____, and _____.**

The chest does not rise and fall with ventilation, the rate is too slow or too fast for the age of the patient, and the heart rate does not return to normal.

○   **What is the most common technique for opening the airway?**

The head-tilt/chin-lift maneuver.

○   **What technique would you use for opening the airway when you suspect spinal injury?**

The jaw-thrust maneuver.

○   **After performing the head-tilt/chin-lift, you note secretions in the patient's oropharynx. What do you do?**

Suction.

○   **What is the purpose of suctioning?**

Remove blood, other liquids and food particles from the airway.

○   **What kinds of things may suctioning prove inadequate to remove?**

Teeth, foreign bodies, food.

○   **You are bagging a patient and hear a gurgling sound with each ventilation. What should you do?**

Suction.

○   **What two types of portable suction devices are there?**

Electrical and hand operated.

○   **What two types of suction catheters are there?**

Hard or rigid (tonsil tip) and soft (French).

○   **How far should you insert a rigid catheter when suctioning?**

Only as far as you can see.

○   **When might you use a soft suction catheter rather than a rigid?**

To suction the nasopharynx, endotracheal tubes.

○   **How far should you insert a soft catheter into the pharynx?**

Only as far as the base of the tongue.

O   **How much vacuum should a suction device be able to generate?**

300 mm Hg.

O   **What is the main disadvantage of a battery operated suction unit?**

Discharged batteries.

O   **T/F: Never insert a suction catheter without suction.**

False.

O   **What is the maximum time you should apply suction to a patient?**

15 seconds at a time.

O   **In infants and children, should this time be shorter or longer?**

Shorter, more specifically, less than 10 seconds; children have less capacity to tolerate hypoxia.

O   **What should you do if the patient has secretions or emesis that cannot be removed quickly and easily by suctioning?**

The patient should be logrolled and the oropharynx should by cleared.

O   **What is the procedure for handling a patient producing frothy secretions as rapidly as suctioning can remove?**

Suction for 15 seconds, ventilate for two minutes, then suction for 15 seconds, and continue in that manner. Consult medical direction for this situation.

O   **You are suctioning a patient and the tubing becomes clogged. What should you do?**

Attempt to clear the clog by suctioning water.

O   **In order of preference, the four methods for ventilating a patient by the rescuer are:**

Mouth-to-mask.
Two-person bag-valve mask.
Flow-restricted, oxygen powered ventilation device.
One person bag-valve mask.

○   **Before beginning artificial ventilations of any kind, what should you consider?**

Body substance isolation.

○   **What oxygen liter flow should you use when performing mouth-to-mask ventilations?**

15L/min.

○   **What are the components of the bag-valve-mask?**

Self-inflating bag, one-way valve, facemask, oxygen reservoir.   To perform most effectively, it needs to be connected to oxygen.

○   **What is the approximate volume of the self-inflating bag?**

1,600 ml.

○   **T/F: The bag-valve mask provides less volume than mouth-to-mask.**

True.

○   **T/F: The single rescuer may have difficulty maintaining an airtight seal.**

True.

○   **T/F: Two rescuers using the bag-valve-mask will be more effective than one.**

True.

○   **T/F: Position self at the side of the patient's head for optimal performance of bag-valve mask.**

False. You should be positioned at the top of the patient's head.

○   **What adjunctive airways may be necessary to effectively ventilate with the bag-valve-mask?**

Oropharyngeal or nasopharyngeal airways.

○   **What characteristics should the self-refilling bag have?**

It should be able to be easily cleaned and sterilized.

○ **What kind of valve should the bag-valve-mask have?**

A non-jam valve that allows a maximum of oxygen inlet flow of 15L/min.

○ **When using two hands to secure a mask for ventilation, which fingers hold the mask down?**

The thumbs.

○ **How often should you repeat ventilations on an adult?**

One ventilation every five seconds.

○ **How often should you repeat ventilations on a child?**

One ventilation every three seconds.

○ **If while ventilating a patient, the chest does not rise and fall, what is the first thing you should do?**

Reposition the head.

○ **If while ventilating a patient the chest does not rise and fall, what should you do after repositioning the head?**

If air is escaping from under the mask, reposition fingers and mask.

○ **If while ventilating a patient the chest does not rise and fall, what should you do after repositioning fingers and mask?**

Check for obstruction.

○ **If while ventilating a patient the chest does not rise and fall, what should you do after checking for obstruction?**

Use alternative method of artificial ventilation, e.g. pocket mask, manually triggered device. If necessary, consider the use of adjuncts such as oral or nasal airways.

○ **What precautions should you take in ventilating a patient with suspected trauma or neck injury?**

Immobilize the head and neck. Have an assistant immobilize, or immobilize between your knees.

O   **What type of ventilatory device is contraindicated in children?**

Oxygen powered ventilation devices.

O   **What peak flow rate and percent of oxygen should a flow-restricted oxygen-powered ventilation device be capable of delivering?**

100% at up to 40L/min.

O   **At what pressure should the inspiratory pressure relief valve activate on a flow-restricted oxygen-powered ventilation device?**

60 cc/water.

O   **In addition to a pressure relief valve, what safety features should a flow-restricted oxygen-powered ventilation device have?**

An audible alarm that sounds whenever the relief-valve pressure is exceeded.

O   **How should the trigger be positioned on a flow-restricted oxygen-powered ventilation device?**

In such a way that both hands can remain on the mask to hold it in position.

O   **What is a tracheostomy?**

A permanent artificial opening in the trachea.

O   **What special procedures do you need to use when ventilating a tracheostomy patient?**

If unable to artificially ventilate, try suction, then artificial ventilation through the nose and mouth; sealing the stoma may improve ability to artificially ventilate from above or may clear obstruction. You need to seal the mouth and nose when air is escaping.

O   **How do you use a bag-valve-mask to stoma?**

Use infant and child mask to make seal. The technique is otherwise very similar to ventilating through the mouth. The head and neck do not need to be positioned.

O   **When may an oropharyngeal airway be used?**

In assisting in maintaining an open airway on unresponsive patients without a gag reflex.

O   **What is the preferred method for inserting an oral airway in an adult?**

Open the mouth, insert the airway upside down, advance until resistance is encountered, then turn the airway 180 degrees so that it comes to rest with the flange on the patient's teeth.

O   **What is the preferred method of inserting an oral airway in a pediatric patient, and an alternative method in an adult?**

Insert the airway right side up, using a tongue depressor to press the tongue down and avoid obstructing the airway.

O   **When may a nasopharyngeal airway be used?**

On patients who are responsive but need assistance keeping the tongue from obstructing the airway. Less noxious than the oral airway.

O   **How do you select the proper size of nasal airway?**

Measure from the tip of the nose to the tip of the patient's ear. Also, consider the diameter of the airway in the nostril.

O   **How do you insert the nasal airway?**

Lubricate the airway with a water-soluble lubricant. Insert it posteriorly. The bevel should be toward the base of the nostril or toward the septum.

O   **What do you do if you are unable to advance a nasal airway?**

Try the other nostril.

O   **What is the capacity of a D cylinder?**

350 L

O   **What is the capacity of an E cylinder?**

625 L

O   **What is the capacity of an M cylinder?**

3,000 L

O   **What is the capacity of a G cylinder?**

5,300 L

O   **What is the capacity of an H cylinder?**

6,900 L

O   **Why is it important to handle oxygen tanks carefully?**

Their contents are under pressure.

O   **What is the most delicate part of the oxygen cylinder?**

The valve and gauge assembly.

O   **What precautions can you take to avoid damaging oxygen cylinders?**

They should be positioned to prevent falling, and secured during transport.

O   **Approximately how many pounds per square inch (PSI) does a full oxygen cylinder hold?**

2000.

O   **When is it important to humidify oxygen?**

If the patient is going to be on it for an extended period.

O   **What two steps must you take before attaching the regulator-flowmeter to the oxygen tank?**

Remove the protective seal and quickly open and then shut the valve.

O   **After using an oxygen tank, what steps should you take to secure the system?**

Close the valve, and bleed remaining oxygen from the regulator.

O   **What is the preferred method of giving oxygen to pre-hospital patients and why?**

Non-rebreathing mask. Delivers up to 90% O2.

O   **What common error is made when placing a non-rebreathing mask on a patient?**

Bag not full before placing mask.

❍   **How do you determine the correct flow rate for the non-rebreather mask?**

When the patient inhales, the bag should not collapse.

❍   **Regarding what types of patients are there unwarranted concerns about giving "too much" oxygen?**

COPD patients and infants. Research has shown that concerns about the dangers of giving these patients too much oxygen are not valid. All patients who require oxygen (are cyanotic, cool, clammy, short of breath) should receive high concentration oxygen.

❍   **When should nasal cannula be used?**

Only when the patient will not tolerate a non-rebreathing mask, despite coaching.

❍   **You arrive at a playground where a six month-old child is being held by her frantic mother. You assess the child and find she is not breathing. In what position do you place this child's head for ventilation?**

In the correct neutral position. This is true for both infants and children from 1-8 years of age.

❍   **What is the correct head position for ventilating a child?**

Extended slightly past neutral.

❍   **Why is it important not to hyperextend the head of an infant or child when ventilating?**

Their trachea and necks are very pliable and you may occlude the airway.

❍   **What special concerns do you have in using the bag-valve-mask on a pediatric patient?**

Avoid excessive bag pressure. Use only enough to make the chest rise; more than that can damage the lungs and inflate the stomach.

❍   **T/F: Gastric distention is more common in adults than in children.**

False.

❍   **If you are unable to ventilate a child using the head tilt, jaw thrust or chin lift, what should you do?**

Consider an oral or nasal airway.

○   **What problems do facial injuries pose to establishing and maintaining a patent airway?**

Because the blood supply to the face is so rich, blunt injuries to the face frequently result in severe swelling. For the same reason, bleeding into the airway from facial injuries can be a challenge to manage.

○   **T/F: Ordinary dentures should always be removed before ventilating a patient.**

False.

○   **What is the concern with partial dentures when ventilating a patient?**

They may become dislodged and occlude the airway.

○   **Identify the following: a leaf shaped structure that prevents food and liquid from entering the trachea during swallowing.**

Epiglottis.

○   **Identify the following: firm cartilage ring forming the lower portion of the larynx.**

Cricoid cartilage.

○   **Identify the following: two major branches of the trachea to the lungs.**

Bronchi.

○   **Describe the active process of inhalation.**

Diaphragm and intercostal muscles contract, increasing the size of the thoracic cavity. Ribs move upward and outward. Air flows into lungs.

○   **Describe the process of air exchange at the alveolar/capillary level.**

Oxygen rich air enters the alveoli during each inspiration. Oxygen poor blood in the capillaries passes into the alveoli. Oxygen enters the capillaries as carbon dioxide enters the alveoli.

○   **Describe the normal respiratory pattern.**

The rate and rhythm is regular, the breathing effort is unlabored, without the use of accessory muscles. Breath sounds are present bilaterally. Chest expansion is adequate and equal.

❍   **List some signs of inadequate breathing.**

Rate is outside normal limits for the age of the patient. Breath sounds are diminished or absent. The respiratory effort is increased with use of accessory muscles. The tidal volume may be inadequate or shallow. Nasal flaring may be present. The skin may be pale or cyanotic and cool and clammy. Agonal breathing may be seen just before death.

❍   **What is the best method for opening an airway?**

Use the head-tilt, chin lift when there is no suspicion of neck injury.

❍   **What are some complications of orotracheal suctioning?**

Cardiac arrhythmia, hypoxia, coughing, mucosal damage and bronchospasm.

❍   **Occasionally you may need to use a technique called the "Sellick Maneuver." Describe this technique and the indications for its use.**

The "Sellick Maneuver" is slight pressure placed on the cricoid cartilage when intubating a patient. The purpose of the maneuver is to prevent passive regurgitation and aspiration during endotracheal intubation, and may also aid in visualizing the vocal cords.

❍   **Where should you look to find the cricoid cartilage?**

To find the cricoid cartilage, the depression below the thyroid cartilage (Adam's apple) is palpated. This corresponds to the cricothyroid membrane.

❍   **What is the purpose of orotracheal intubation?**

It is the most effective means of controlling a patient's airway. It is used in apneic patients. It provides good control of the airway and minimizes risk of aspiration. It allows for better oxygen delivery and deeper suctioning.

❍   **Describe the possible complications that may result from orotracheal intubation.**

A slowing of the heart rate may occur as a result of stimulating the airway. It may cause damage to the lips, teeth, gums and airway structures. It may cause vomiting, esophageal intubation, and right main-stem bronchus intubation.

❍   **Assorted sizes of endotracheal tubes are available for patient use. What size of ET tube should you place in an adult male?**

8.0 – 8.5 mm.

○ **Assorted sizes of endotracheal tubes are available for patient use. What size of ET tube should you place in an adult female?**

7.0 – 8.0 mm.

○ **Assorted sizes of endotracheal tubes are available for patient use. If limited equipment is available, what size of ET tube could be used in an emergency?**

7.5 fits any adult in an emergency.

○ **Describe the components of an endotracheal tube and their functions.**

15-mm adapter --allows for attachment of bag-valve-mask.
Pilot balloon – verifies the cuff is inflated.
Cuff – holds approximately 10cc of air to provide a seal.

○ **What is the maximum age of a patient in which an uncuffed ET tube is used.**

Eight years old.

○ **What is the average distance from the teeth to the vocal cords?**

15 centimeters.

○ **What is the average distance from the teeth to the sternal notch?**

20 centimeters.

○ **What is the average distance from the teeth to the carina?**

25 centimeters.

○ **What device can be used to help shape the ET tube?**

A stylet.

○ **How far should a stylet be inserted into the ET tube?**

A stylet should be inserted to, but not beyond, the Murphy's eye.

○ **Identify several indications for intubation.**

The inability to ventilate an apneic patient; patient with no gag reflex; the inability of the patient to protect his own airway, e.g., cardiac arrest, unresponsiveness.

❍ **Elena, working the Combat Zone, is responding to a report of "an unconscious person who fell from a rooftop." What should she keep in mind when intubating this patient?**

If trauma is suspected, the patient must be intubated with the head and neck in a neutral position using in-line stabilization.

❍ **Antonio is preparing to intubate a cardiac arrest patient. What is the proper landmark he should use for insertion of a curved blade laryngoscope?**
The curved blade should be inserted into the vallecula and lifted upward.

❍ **Sam is preparing to intubate an overdose patient. What is the proper landmark he should use for insertion of a straight blade laryngoscope?**

The straight blade is used to directly lift the epiglottis, then insert the ET tube.

❍ **Ensuring proper placement of the ET tube is absolutely essential. Describe the technique that Captain Veronica, the senior EMT, should use after intubating a trauma patient to ensure proper tube placement.**

Auscultate breath sounds, begin over the epigastrium. No sounds should be heard during artificial respiration. Listen over the left apex; compare with the right apex. Breath sounds should be heard bilaterally.

❍ **Your Lieutenant, Jacob, has just intubated a patient. While assessing breath sounds for him, you notice they are slightly diminished on the left side of the chest. What does this finding indicate?**

If breath sounds are diminished or absent on the left, most likely a right main-stem bronchus intubation has occurred.

❍ **Why must there be no pop-off (or a disabled pop-off) valve on the bag-valve mask?**

It may result in inadequate ventilation.

❍ **What is the purpose of the oxygen reservoir?**

The oxygen reservoir allows for a higher concentration of oxygen.

❍ **What sizes of masks should you carry for the bag-valve-mask?**

Infant, child and adult.

○   **Where should you position the apex of the mask of the bag-valve-mask?**

Over the patient's nose.

○   **When using two hands to secure a mask for ventilation, which fingers hold the mask down?**

The thumbs.

○   **When using one hand to secure a mask for ventilation, which fingers hold the mask down?**
The thumb and index fingers.

○   **What is the preferred method for inserting an oral airway in an adult?**

Open the mouth, insert the airway upside down, advance until resistance is encountered, then turn the airway 180 degrees so that it comes to rest with the flange on the patient's teeth.

○   **What is the preferred method of inserting an oral airway in a pediatric patient, and an alternative method in an adult?**

Insert the airway right side up, using a tongue depressor to press the tongue down and avoid obstructing the airway.

○   **When may a nasopharyngeal airway be used?**

On patients who are responsive but need assistance keeping the tongue from obstructing the airway. Less noxious than the oral airway.

○   **What is the preferred method of giving oxygen to prehospital patients and why?**

Nonrebreathing mask. Delivers up to 90% O2.

○   **What common error is made when placing a nonrebreathing mask on a patient?**

Bag not full before placing mask.

○   **How do you determine the correct flow rate for the nonrebreathing mask?**

When the patient inhales, the bag should not collapse.

○   **Regarding what types of patients are there unwarranted concerns about giving "too much" oxygen?**

COPD patients and infants.

○   **What does research indicate in regard to the administration of high concentrations of oxygen to COPD patients and infants in the prehospital setting?**

Research has shown that concerns about the dangers of giving these patients too much oxygen are not valysm, acute pericarditis, previous allergic reaction to thrombolytic agents, and severe persistent hypertension with a systolic greater than 180 mmHg or diastolic greater than 110 mmHg.

○   **The pharynx is composed of what two structures?**

The oropharynx and the nasopharynx.

○   **What is the function of the epiglottis?**

The epiglottis prevents food and liquid from entering the trachea during swallowing.

○   **What is the windpipe called?**

The trachea.

○   **Where is the cricoid cartilage located?**

The cricoid cartilage is a firm cartilaginous ring forming the lower portion of the larynx.

○   **What is the voice box called?**

The larynx.

○   **What are the bronchi?**

The bronchi are the two major branches of the trachea to the lungs. Each bronchus subdivides into smaller air passages called the bronchioles, which end at the alveoli.

○   **What muscles contract during inhalation?**

The diaphragm and the intercostal muscles.

○   **What are the three basic steps of alveolar/capillary exchange?**

Oxygen-rich air enters the alveoli during each inspiration.
Oxygen-poor blood in the capillaries passes into the walls of the alveoli.

Oxygen enters the capillaries as carbon dioxide enters the alveoli.

O   **What are the two basic components of the capillary/cellular exchange in the alveoli?**

Cells give up carbon dioxide to the capillaries.
Capillaries give up oxygen to the cells.

O   **What is the normal breathing rate for an adult?**

12-20 breaths per minute.

O   **What is the normal breathing rate for a child?**

15-30 breaths per minute.

O   **What is the normal breathing rate for an infant?**

25-50 breaths per minute.

O   **Which two words are used to describe basic breathing rhythm?**

Regular and irregular.

O   **How would you describe normal breath sounds?**

Present and equal.

O   **How would you describe normal chest expansion?**

Adequate and equal.

O   **How would you describe increased effort of breathing?**

Use of accessory muscles, predominantly in infants and children.

O   **How would you describe normal depth of breathing?**

Adequate.

ARRHYTHMIAS, DEFIBRILLATION, AND PACING

○ **What is the normal duration of the P-R interval?**

0.12 to 0.20 seconds.

○ **What will NOT occur during the absolute refractory period?**

Cardiac cells cannot be stimulated to depolarize. The absolute refractory period occurs from the onset of the QRS complex to approximately the peak of the T wave.

○ **What are the key characteristics of first degree A-V block?**

- Atrial and ventricular rates are the same.
- The atrial and ventricular rhythm is regular.
- The P waves are normal in size and configuration with one P wave before each QRS complex.
- The P-R interval is prolonged greater than 0.20 seconds but is constant.
- The QRS is usually 0.10 seconds or less in duration.

○ **What are the characteristics of second degree A-V block Mobitz Type I?**

- Atrial rate is greater than ventricular rate.
- Atrial rhythm is regular, ventricular rate is irregular.
- P waves are normal in size and configuration, however, not all P waves are followed by a QRS.
- The P-R interval lengthens with each cycle until a P wave appears without a QRS.
- The QRS interval is generally 0.10 seconds or less in duration and is dropped periodically.

○ **What valve separates the right ventricle from the right atrium?**

The tricuspid valve.

○   **What is the following rhythm?**

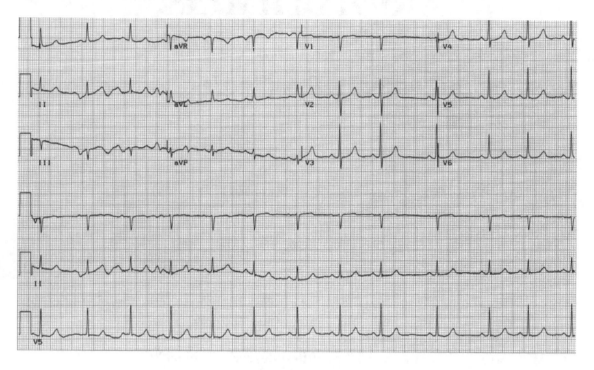

Sinus arrhythmia.

○   **Where is the sinoatrial node located?**

Junction of the superior vena cava and the right atrium.

○   **What is the inherent rate of an idioventricular rhythm?**

20 - 40 beats per minute.

○   **What are the key features of atrial flutter?**

- Atrial rate 250 - 350 beats per minute, ventricular rate is variable.
- Atrial rhythm is regular and ventricular rhythm may be regular or irregular.
- P waves, flutter waves (saw-toothed).
- P-R interval not measurable.
- QRS generally 0.10 seconds in duration or less, but may be greater if aberrantly conducted.
- QRS widening may occur if flutter waves are buried in the QRS complex.

○   **What is the first positive deflection seen after the P wave on the ECG?**

The R wave.

○ **What is the following rhythm?**

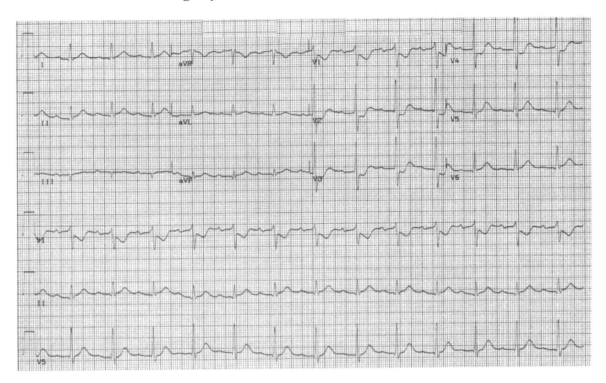

A sinus rhythm with depressed S-T segments and inverted T waves.

○ **What is the following rhythm?**

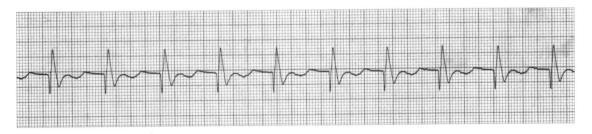

100% ventricular paced rhythm. Spikes are present before each QRS complex.

○ **Identify the relative refractory period on an ECG.**

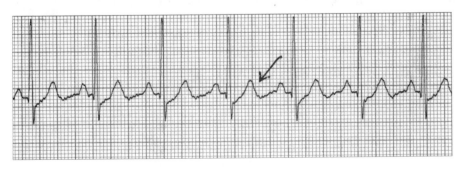

The down slope of the T wave. During this period, it is possible to stimulate the cardiac cells to depolarize, which may precipitate V-tach or V-fib.

○   **What is located at the A-V junction?**

The A-V node and the non-branching portion of the Bundle of His.

○   **What occurs during the QRS complex?**

Ventricular depolarization.

○   **How is the P-R interval measured?**

From the beginning of the P wave to the beginning of the QRS complex.

○   **How is the Q-T interval measured?**

From the beginning of the QRS complex to the end of the T wave.

○   **T/F: The Q-T interval represents the time required for ventricular depolarization and repolarization.**

True.

○   **Contrast a junctional escape rhythm from that of a ventricular escape rhythm.**

A junctional rhythm is supraventricular in origin and the QRS complex will be 0.10 seconds or less. Ventricular escape rhythms are derived from the ventricles and will have a wide QRS complex greater than 0.12 seconds.

○   **Trace the normal electrical flow through the heart.**

S-A node to the A-V node, then to the Bundle of His where it is divided into the left and right bundle branches, and then to the Purkinje fibers where mechanical cells are stimulated.

○   **What is the inherent rate of the A-V junctional or nodal rhythm.**

40 - 60 beats per minute.

○   **What are the key features of third degree A-V block?**

- P waves occur regularly and there are more P waves than QRS complexes.
- The ventricular rhythm is regular.
- The atria and ventricles beat independently of each other.

- The QRS may be narrow or wide depending on the location of the escape pacemaker.

○ **What is the normal rate of sinus tachycardia?**

Greater than 100 beats per minute.

○ **What is the normal duration of the QRS complex in an adult?**

0.04 to 0.1 seconds.

○ **Contrast second degree A-V block, Mobitz Type I and second degree A-V block, Mobitz Type II.**

In second degree A-V block Mobitz Type I, the P-R interval lengthens until a P wave appears without a QRS complex; in second degree A-V block Mobitz Type II, the P-R interval remains constant until a P wave appears with a dropped QRS.

○ **Where is the conduction defect located in second degree A-V block, Mobitz Type I?**

A-V node.

○ **Where is the conduction defect located in second degree A-V block, Mobitz Type II?**

At or below the Bundle of His.

○ **What is the differential diagnosis of sinus tachycardia?**

Volume depletion, pain, stress, fever, pump failure, hypoxia, or shock.

○ **What are the key features of second degree A-V block with 2 to 1 conduction?**

- P waves occur regularly with more P waves than QRS complexes, every other P wave is followed by a QRS complex.
- Constant P-P interval, dropped QRS every other beat.
- QRS may be narrow or wide.

❍   **What is the following rhythm?**

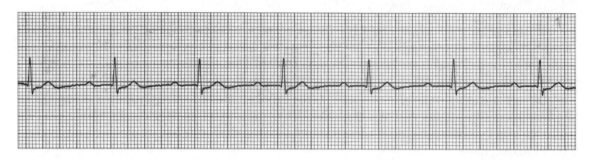

First degree A-V block.

❍   **What is the following rhythm?**

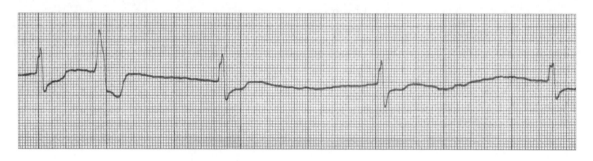

Idioventricular rhythm. Features include:
- Atrial rate is not discernible, whereas the ventricular rate is 20-40 beats per minute.
- Ventricular rhythm is essentially regular.
- P waves are absent or retrograde, QRS is greater than 0.12 seconds.

❍   **Contrast second degree A-V block, Mobitz Type I from third degree A-V block.**

In second degree A-V block, type I, the atrial rhythm is regular, the ventricular rhythm is irregular, and the P-R interval lengthens until a P wave appears with no QRS complex. In third-degree A-V block, the atrial and ventricular rhythms are regular and there is no P-R interval since the atria and ventricles beat independently of each other. Furthermore, the atrial rate is approximately twice the ventricular rate.

❍   **What are alternative names for second degree A-V block, type I?**

Mobitz Type I or Wenckebach.

❍   **What is the following rhythm?**

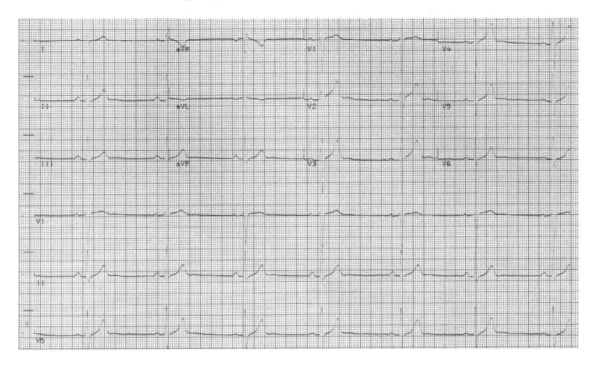

Sinus bradycardia. Key features include:
- A rate of less than 60 beats per minute.
- Atrial and ventricular rhythms are regular.
- P waves are uniform and upright with one P wave before each QRS complex.
- P-R interval is 0.12 to 0.20 seconds.

QRS is usually 0.10 seconds or less.

❍   **What is the differential diagnosis of premature atrial complexes?**

Digitalis toxicity, congestive heart failure, myocardial injury, sympathomimetic drugs, hypoxia, and stimulants.

❍   **What is the following rhythm?**

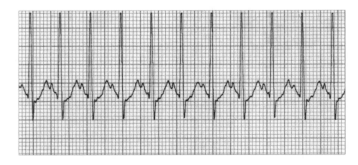

Sinus tachycardia. Key characteristics include:

- A rate of 100-160 bpm.
- A regular rhythm.
- Upright P waves with one preceding each QRS complex.
- P-R interval of 0.12 to 0.20 seconds.
- 0.10 second QRS duration or less.

○ **What is the following dysrhythmia?**

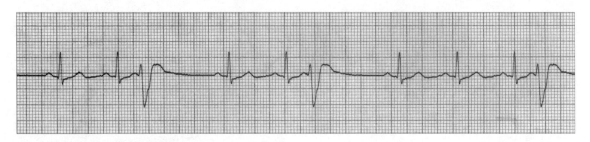

Sinus rhythm with frequent premature ventricular complexes.

○ **What is the differential diagnosis of a flatline on an ECG monitor?**

Asystole, isoelectric V-fib/V-tach, failed connection, no power, and loose leads.

○ **What are the indications for unsynchronized countershock?**

Pulseless ventricular tachycardia, ventricular fibrillation, sustained Torsades de Pointes, and ventricular tachycardia with a pulse if the clinical condition has deteriorated.

○ **What energy level is used to treat an unstable patient with atrial flutter?**

Synchronized countershock with 50, 100, 200, 300, and 360 joules.

○ **What is the electrical treatment for an unstable patient with ventricular tachycardia?**

100, 200, 300, and 360 joules.

○ **What are the most common complications of transcutaneous pacing?**

Skin burns, pain, coughing, and interference with sensing as a result of patient agitation or muscle contractions.

○ **How do you confirm asystole with quick look paddles?**

Check by positioning the paddles for lead 2 then rotate the paddles 90 degrees to simulate placement for lead 1 or lead 3.

○ **What is the electrical therapy for an unstable patient with atrial fibrillation?**

Synchronized countershock at 100, 200, 300, and 360 joules.

○ **What is the distance that defibrillation paddles must be placed from a pacemaker?**

At least five inches.

○ **Why shock first in ventricular fibrillation or pulseless ventricular tachycardia?**

Electroshock therapy is more important than drug therapy in the treatment of ventricular fibrillation and pulseless ventricular tachycardia.

○ **What are the indications for transcutaneous pacing?**

Bradycardia with unstable vital signs unresponsive to pharmacological therapy, asystolic cardiac arrest, overdrive pacing of SVT.

○ **Describe the various types of vagal maneuvers.**

Carotid sinus pressure, coughing, eyeball pressure, breath holding, facial immersion in ice water, valsalva, and gag reflex stimulation.

○ **What is the effect of a vagal maneuver?**

Vagal maneuvers slow conduction through the AV node by increasing parasympathetic tone.

○ **Describe the placement of defibrillation paddles.**

The sternum paddle is placed just to the right of the upper sternum and below the clavicle and the apex paddle is placed in the mid-axillary line just to the left of the nipple.

○ **What are the complications of carotid sinus pressure?**

Ventricular dysrhythmias, bradycardia, seizures, syncope, and CVA.

○ **What is the level of shock therapy recommended for paroxysmal supraventricular tachycardia?**

Synchronized countershock at 50, 100, 200, 300, and 360 joules.

○ **What are the contraindications to transcutaneous pacing?**

Chest trauma, barrel chest, weight less than 15 kg, and cervical spine injury. Transcutaneous pacing may be used if pediatric pacing beds are available.

○   **Explain the difference between defibrillation and synchronized countershock.**

Defibrillation, also known as unsynchronized countershock, has no relationship to the cardiac cycle whereas a synchronized countershock is delivered a few milliseconds after the peak of the R wave.

○   **Why use synchronized shock?**

Reduces the risk of delivering the shock during the vulnerable period of the T wave.

○   **Why must transdermal nitroglycerin patches be removed prior to delivering countershock?**

Transdermal patches may lead to electrical arcing, resulting in smoke, burns, explosive noises, and paired delivery of current.

○   **In a 30-kg child, what would be the initial energy level for defibrillation?**

60 J.

○   **In an adult, what is the initial energy level used to defibrillate ventricular fibrillation?**

200 J.

○   **What factors decrease resistance to transthoracic flow of a defibrillating current?**

Use of a conductive medium, successive countershocks, and lower patient body weight.

○   **In what two situations is synchronized cardioversion indicated?**

Symptomatic supraventricular tachycardia and symptomatic ventricular tachycardia.

○   **CPR is in progress in an unwitnessed cardiac arrest in which ventricular fibrillation is present on the monitor. What should be the first treatment?**

Defibrillate with 200 J of unsynchronized electricity.

○   **T/F: Synchronized countershock is indicated for unstable patients with polymorphic ventricular tachycardia.**

False. Use unsynchronized countershock.

○   **What are the indications for procainamide administration?**

Procainamide is used when lidocaine has failed to suppress ventricular ectopy. Procainamide is typically used in refractory or pulseless ventricular tachycardia or ventricular fibrillation. It may also be used in atrial fibrillation with a rapid ventricular response and wide complex tachycardia that cannot be distinguished from ventricular tachycardia.

○   **What is chronotropy?**

Chronotropy refers to heart rate effect. A positive chronotropic effect refers to an increase in the heart rate whereas a negative chronotropic effect refers to a decrease in the heart rate.

○   **What is the dose of calcium chloride?**

2-4 mg/kg of a 10% solution. Note: Calcium should be administered slowly.

○   **How is adenosine administered?**

It is administered in a single, large bolus. Generally 6 mg rapid IV bolus over 1-3 seconds followed by a 20 ml saline flush.

○   **What is the effect of dobutamine infused at a rate of 5 mcg/kg/min?**

Increased cardiac output, increased myocardial contractility, and increased myocardial oxygen requirements.

○   **What is the effect of digitalis on the heart?**

Increases myocardial contractility and slows the heart rate by decreasing conduction through the AV node.

○   **What is the effect of verapamil on myocardial contraction?**

Verapamil is a calcium channel blocker, which decreases the force of myocardial contractions.

○   **What are the signs and symptoms of magnesium overdose?**

Flushing, hypotension, bradycardia, AV block, respiratory depression, sweating, drowsiness, decreased consciousness, diminished reflexes, and flaccid paralysis.

❍   **What are possible effects of magnesium sulfate?**

It is thought that magnesium sulfate may decrease the incidence of acute myocardial infarction mortality due to improved myocardial metabolism, coronary vasodilatation, decreased myocardial infarct size, decreased platelet aggregation, systemic vasodilatation, and protection against catecholamine-induced myocardial necrosis.

❍   **What is the mechanism of action of sodium nitroprusside?**

Peripheral vasodilatation of both the arterial and venous systems resulting in increased cardiac output, and decreased preload, afterload, and myocardial oxygen requirements.

❍   **What is the typical starting dose of norepinephrine?**

0.15-30 mcg/min.

❍   **What is the indication for norepinephrine administration?**

Cardiogenic shock and severe hypotension.

❍   **What is the correct dose of sodium bicarbonate?**

1 mEq/kg.

❍   **During cardiac arrest, when is sodium bicarbonate administration most strongly indicated?**

In pre-existing hyperkalemia.

❍   **What is the correct dose of magnesium sulfate in a patient with Torsades de Pointes?**

1-2 g IV bolus.

❍   **What is the benefit of epinephrine during cardiac arrest?**

Epinephrine provides alpha adrenergic receptor stimulation resulting in peripheral vasoconstriction. Peripheral vasoconstriction improves coronary and cerebral blood flow.

❍   **What drugs are used to treat narrow QRS tachycardia?**

Adenosine, verapamil, beta-blockers, digoxin, and diltiazem.

❍   **What are the indications for the use of diltiazem?**

Atrial flutter, atrial fibrillation with a rapid ventricular response, and multifocal atrial tachycardia.

○ **What are the effects of norepinephrine?**

Alpha and beta-adrenergic receptor-stimulating properties. The effects include increased heart rate, increased myocardial contractility, peripheral vasoconstriction and renal and mesenteric constriction.

○ **T/F: Dopamine is the drug of choice for the treatment of heart failure when the systolic blood pressure is less than 90 mmHg.**

True. Dopamine increases myocardial contractility and as a result increases cardiac output.

○ **T/F: Epinephrine is the first drug used in the treatment of asystole, ventricular fibrillation, pulseless ventricular tachycardia, and pulseless electrical activity.**

True.

○ **In what condition should beta-blockers be avoided?**

Profound bradycardia, second or third degree AV block, hypotension, congestive heart failure, and bronchospastic disease.

○ **What is the correct dose of lidocaine?**

1-1.5 mg/kg bolus, which is then, repeated at 1/2 the initial dose every 5-10 minutes to a total of 3 mg/kg.

○ **What are the most common side effects of bretylium?**

Nausea, vomiting, and hypotension.

○ **What ECG findings should be monitored during procainamide administration?**

Watch for increasing P-R intervals, increasing Q-T intervals, and widening QRS complex.

○ **What is an extremely dangerous complication of procainamide administration?**

Torsades de Pointes.

○ **What is the most frequent complication of thrombolytic therapy?**

Bleeding. Hypotension may also occur with streptokinase administration.

○ **What are the symptoms of digitalis toxicity?**

Blurred vision, changes in color perception, fatigue, nausea, vomiting, decreased appetite, diarrhea, dizziness, headache, abnormal dreaming, weakness, sinus arrest, blocks, and atrial and ventricular tachycardia.

○ **What are the side effects of beta-blockers?**

Bradycardia, hypotension, bronchospasm, and precipitation of congestive heart failure.

○ **What are the side effects of isoproterenol administration?**

Tachycardia, palpitations, dysrhythmias, hypertension, angina, MI extension, anxiety, insomnia, nervousness, dizziness, tremor, weakness, headache, and nausea, vomiting, sweating, and flushing of the face or skin.

IV ACCESS, RESUSCITATION, CIRCULATION, AND MONITORING

❍ **What are the common complications of IV therapy?**

Cellulitis, thrombosis, phlebitis, infiltration, and hematoma formation.

❍ **What is the IV site of choice in an acute cardiac arrest?**

The antecubital vein or as a second choice, the internal jugular vein.

❍ **What IV solution should be used during a cardiac arrest?**

Normal saline or lactated ringers.

❍ **What are the systemic complications of IV therapy?**

Air embolism, sepsis, pulmonary thromboembolism, circulatory overload, and catheter fragmentation embolism.

❍ **What are the complications of subclavian or internal jugular venipuncture?**

Air embolism, dysrhythmias, hemothorax, infiltration into the pleural space or mediastinum, and pneumothorax.

❍ **What are the advantages of peripheral venipuncture over central venous access?**

Peripheral venipuncture is easier, quicker, avoids interruption of CPR, and has a lower complication rate.

❍ **What are the indications for central venous access?**

Immediate access to venous circulation, administration of irritating solutions, elevation of central venous pressure, and passage of catheters into the pulmonary and cardiac circulation.

❍   **What are the advantages of femoral vein cannulation during CPR?**

Avoids interruption of CPR, provides easy access to the central circulation, and it does not easily collapse like peripheral veins, no risk of pneumothorax.

❍   **A 4 year-old is found by paramedics in acute cardiac arrest. An IV cannot be started. How should epinephrine be given?**

Intraosseous route or endotracheal route.

❍   **In an infant, what type of fluid bolus should be used?**

Lactated Ringer's solution, 20 cc/kg.

❍   **What vein is the most suitable for cannulation during external cardiac compression?**

The antecubital vein.

❍   **What are the most common complications seen in catheter-through-needle systems?**

Infection, shearing of the end of the catheter, and extravasation of infused fluid.

❍   **T/F: Intracardiac injection of drugs is the preferred route during an acute cardiac arrest.**

False. The IV route is preferred.

❍   **What is the key to successful resuscitation of a near drowning victim?**

Ventilatory support.

❍   **What is the major complication from a lightning strike?**

DC countershock and acute respiratory arrest.

❍   **When should an intravenous line established during CPR be replaced?**

After three days.

❍   **What is the focus of the primary survey?**

Airway, Breathing, Circulation, and Defibrillation.

❍   **What is the focus of the secondary survey?**

Intubation, IV access, rhythms, and drug treatment.

❍   **What should be done just prior to performing the primary survey?**

Assess responsiveness, call for help, and position the victim and rescuer.

❍   **What is the order of action for a single rescuer with access to a defibrillator?**

Assess responsiveness, call for help, open airway, give two breaths and check for obstruction, confirm pulselessness, then defibrillate. Note: this sequence omits starting chest compressions.

❍   **What IV fluid is recommended during ACLS?**

Normal saline

❍   **What ACLS drugs can be administered down the endotracheal tube?**

Atropine, lidocaine, and epinephrine.

❍   **What is the dose of medication used via endotracheal tube?**

2 to 2.5 times the normal dose followed by 10 ml of normal saline.

❍   **The artery which is palpable at the top of the foot is called the _____.**

Dorsalis pedis.

❍   **The ratio of compressions to ventilations in adult two-rescuer CPR is _____:_____.**

5:1.

❍   **Gastric distention during CPR is caused by _____.**

Air entering the patient's stomach.

❍   **Describe the importance of automated external defibrillation.**

Successful resuscitation of out-of-hospital arrest depends on a series of critical interventions known as the chain of survival. AED is the third element in the chain.

O   **Identify the components of the chain of survival.**

The components of the American Heart Association chain of survival are early access, early CPR, early defibrillation, and early ACLS.

O   **Describe the rationale for early defibrillation basic in the pre-hospital setting.**

Many EMS systems have demonstrated increased survival outcomes of cardiac arrest patients experiencing ventricular fibrillation when early defibrillation is used in the pre-hospital setting.

O   **Identify a major factor attributed to the increase in survival of cardiac arrest patients in the pre-hospital setting.**

The increased survival of cardiac arrest patients in the pre-hospital setting was directly attributed to early defibrillation programs that were implemented when all the links in the chain of survival were present.

O   **Identify the features of a fully automated external defibrillator.**

A fully automated external defibrillator operates without action by rescuers, except to turn the power on. All operations of the unit are contained within the apparatus and no intervention is needed.

O   **Describe the features of a semi-automated external defibrillator.**

A semi-automated external defibrillator uses a computer voice synthesizer to advise the rescuer of the steps to take based upon the AED's analysis of the patient's cardiac rhythm.

O   **Describe how an AED analyzes the cardiac rhythms of a patient.**

The AED computer microprocessor evaluates the patient's rhythm and confirms the presence of a rhythm for which a shock is indicated. Accuracy of these devices in rhythm analysis has been high, both in detecting rhythms needing defibrillation and rhythms that do not need defibrillation. The analysis is dependent on properly charged defibrillator batteries.

O   **Indicate two reasons the AED may inappropriately deliver shocks.**

Human error and mechanical error.

O   **Identify the proper criteria for attaching the AED to a cardiac patient.**

Attach the defibrillator AED only to unresponsive, pulseless, non-breathing patients to avoid delivering inappropriate shocks.

○   **When properly using an AED in a cardiac arrest patient, the interruption of CPR is necessary. Identify the criteria for which CPR should be interrupted.**

No CPR is performed at times when defibrillations are delivered. No person should be touching the patient when the rhythm is being analyzed and when defibrillations are being delivered. Cardiac compressions and artificial ventilations are stopped when the rhythm is being analyzed and when more defibrillations are delivered. Defibrillation is more effective than CPR, so stopping CPR during the process is more beneficial to the patient outcome.

○   **How long may CPR be interrupted at any given time?**

CPR may be stopped up to 90 seconds if three defibrillations are necessary. Resume CPR only after up to the first three defibrillations are delivered.

○   **You should be able to describe several advantages of automated external defibrillation. Identify those advantages.**

The use of the AED is easier to learn than CPR; however, you must memorize the treatment sequence. Secondly, the EMS delivery system should have all the necessary links in the Chain of Survival. There should be medical direction indicating the proper use of the AED. The first defibrillation should be delivered within one minute of the arrival of the unit at the patient's side.

○   **Identify each of the operational steps necessary to begin using the AED in an unconscious, unresponsive patient.**

Take infection control precautions en route to the incident.
Arrive on scene and perform initial assessment to include ABCs.
Stop CPR if in progress.
Verify pulselessness and apnea.
Have your partner resume CPR.
Attach the AED device.
Turn on defibrillator power.
If the machine has a tape recorder, begin your narrative at this time.
Stop CPR.
Clear the patient and initiate the analysis of the patient.

○   **Identify the proper procedure that should be used if the AED advises defibrillation.**

Deliver the initial defibrillation. The machine will then reanalyze the rhythm. If the machine advises defibrillation, deliver the second shock. Again, the machine will reanalyze the rhythm. If the machine advises a defibrillation, administer the third shock.

At this time, check the patient's pulse. If there is a pulse, check breathing. If breathing adequately, give high concentration of oxygen by non re-breather mask and transport. If not breathing, adequately artificially ventilate the patient with high flow oxygen and transport immediately. If there is no pulse, resume CPR for one minute. Repeat one cycle of up to three stacked defibrillations and transport.

O **Identify when the patient should be transported, assuming no ALS intervention is available on scene.**

The patient should be transported when one of the following occurs: the patient regains a pulse; six defibrillations are delivered; or the machine gives three consecutive messages separated by one minute of CPR, but no defibrillation is advised.

O **After completing an assessment of the ABCs, describe all treatments that precede defibrillation in the pre-hospital setting.**

Following assessment of the ABCs, defibrillation comes first. Do not hook up oxygen or perform any other procedure that delay analysis of rhythm or defibrillation.

O **The rescuer must be familiar with the AED device used in his or her operational EMS setting. Identify several universal procedures that are important for the rescuer basic to understand prior to implementing the use of this device.**

All contact with the patient must be avoided during the analysis of the rhythm. State, "Clear the patient" before delivering any shocks. No defibrillator is capable of working without properly functioning batteries. Check all batteries at the beginning of the shift. It is advisable to carry extra batteries with you.

O **Identify the age and weight guideline when using the AED.**

Automated external defibrillation is not used in cardiac arrest in children under 12 years of age or under 90 lbs. of weight.

O **T/F: Automated external defibrillators can analyze rhythms when the emergency vehicle is in motion.**

False. Automated external defibrillators cannot analyze rhythms when the emergency vehicle is in motion. The vehicle must completely stop in order to analyze rhythm before shocks are ordered. Additionally, it is not safe to defibrillate in a moving ambulance.

O **Identify the most frequent reason for AED defibrillator failure.**

AED defibrillator failure is most frequently related to improper device maintenance, commonly battery failure. Rescuer basics must ensure proper battery maintenance and battery replacement schedules.

○ **Does successful completion of AED training in an EMT basic course permit usage of the device without the approval of state laws, rules, and local medical direction authority?**

No.

○ **Identify several contraindications in giving a patient a nitroglycerin pill.**

A patient should not be given nitroglycerin if they have hypotension or blood pressure below 100 mmHg systolic, or a major head injury. Additionally, nitroglycerin should not be given to infants and children, and patients who have already met the maximum prescribed dose prior to the rescuer arrival. The maximum prescribed dose is one tablet every five minutes up to a maximum of three tablets.

○ **What are the four chambers of the heart?**

Right and left atria, right and left ventricles.

○ **What is the function of the heart valves?**

Valves prevent the backflow of blood into the chamber from where it came.

○ **What does the right atrium do?**

The right atrium receives blood from the veins of the body and the heart, and pumps this deoxygenated blood to the right ventricle.

○ **What does the right ventricle do?**

The right ventricle pumps deoxygenated blood to the lungs.

○ **What does the left atrium do?**

The left atrium receives oxygenated blood from the lungs via the pulmonary veins, and pumps it to the left ventricle.

○ **What does the left ventricle do?**

The left ventricle receives oxygenated blood from the left atrium and pumps it to the body.

○ **What is unique about cardiac muscle?**

It is made up of special contractile and conductive tissue.

❍   **What is the function of the arteries?**

The function of the arteries is to carry oxygenated blood from the heart to the rest of the body.

❍   **What are the arteries of the heart called?**

The coronary arteries.

❍   **What is the function of the coronary arteries?**

The coronary arteries are the vessels that supply the heart with blood.

❍   **What is the major artery originating from the heart?**

The aorta.

❍   **Trace the route taken by the aorta.**

The aorta originates from the left ventricle, and descends anterior to the spine into the thoracic and abdominal cavities. It divides at the level of the pelvic crest into the iliac arteries.

❍   **What is the origin and function of the pulmonary artery?**

The pulmonary artery originates in the right ventricle and carries deoxygenated blood to the lungs.

❍   **What is the function of the carotid arteries?**

Carry oxygenated blood to the head.

❍   **What is the major artery of the thigh?**

The femoral artery.

❍   **Where can you palpate the femoral artery?**

In the crease between the abdomen and the thigh.

❍   **Which vessel supplies the lower arm?**

The radial artery.

○   **Where can you palpate the radial artery?**

Pulsations can be palpated at the wrist, just proximal to the thumb.

○   **Which artery supplies the upper arm?**

The brachial artery.

○   **Where can you palpate the brachial artery?**

Pulsations can be palpated on the inner half of the antecubital fossa at the level of the elbow.

○   **What is another name for a blood pressure cuff?**

Sphygnomanometer.

○   **Which vessel is auscultated when taking a blood pressure?**

The brachial artery.

○   **What is the major vessel supplying the foot?**

The posterior tibial artery.

○   **Where can the posterior tibial artery be palpated?**

On the posterior surface of the medial malleolus.

○   **After the application of a traction splint, how do you evaluate distal circulation and where?**

Palpate the dorsalis pedis on the anterior surface of the foot. Check capillary refill time, sensation, skin condition, and movement.

○   **What is the smallest branch of an artery?**

An arteriole.

○   **What structure connects arterioles and venules?**

Capillaries.

○ **Where are capillaries found?**

In all parts of the body.

○   **You arrive on scene at a restaurant kitchen where you have been called for a man bleeding. When you arrive you find a conscious alert and oriented 45 year-old who states he cut his hand with a knife. You observe dark red blood oozing slowly from a five-centimeter laceration on the palm of his left hand. From what type of blood vessel(s) do you suspect is the source of the bleeding?**

Capillaries.

○   **What is the function of the capillaries?**

They allow for the exchange of nutrients and waste at the cellular level.

○   **What is the smallest branch of the venous system?**

The venules.

○   **What is the function of the venous system?**

To carry deoxygenated blood back to the heart and lungs.

○   **What is the function of the pulmonary vein?**

To carry blood from the lungs to the left atrium.

○   **Why may the pulmonary vein be considered an artery?**

Because it carries oxygenated rather than deoxygenated blood.

○   **What are largest vessels in the venous system?**

The vena cava.

○   **Name the two portions of the vena cava.**

The superior and inferior vena cava.

○   **What is the terminus of the vena cava?**

The right atrium.

○   **What are the four components of blood?**

Red blood cells, white blood cells, plasma and platelets.

○ **What are the two primary functions of the red blood cells?**

To carry oxygen to and carbon dioxide from the organs.

○   **What are the four primary sites for palpating a peripheral pulse on an adult?**

The radial, brachial, posterior tibial and dorsalis pedis arteries.

○   **What are the two primary sites for palpating a central pulse?**

The carotid and femoral arteries.

○   **What causes systolic blood pressure?**

The pressure exerted against the walls of the artery when the left ventricle contracts.

○   **What causes diastolic blood pressure?**

The pressure exerted against the walls of the artery when the left ventricle is at rest.

○   **What is hypoperfusion?**

Inadequate circulation, shock.

○   **You auscultate a blood pressure of 80/60, and take an axillary temperature of 34 degrees C. Are these normal findings given the patient's condition?**

Low or decreasing blood pressure (hypotension) and subnormal temperature are both signs of late, decompensated shock.

○   **What is the definition of perfusion?**

Perfusion is the circulation of blood through an organ or a structure.

○   **What is the function of perfusion?**

The delivery of oxygen and other nutrients to the cells of all organ systems and the removal of waste products.

○   **What is hypoperfusion?**

The inadequate circulation of blood through an organ or a structure.

○   **What are the three types of muscle?**

Voluntary (skeletal), involuntary (smooth), cardiac.

○   **Which muscles are responsible for movement?**

Skeletal.

○   **Which muscles are responsible for carrying out automatic muscular functions?**

Smooth.

○   **Which muscles are under the control of the brain and nervous system?**

Skeletal.

○   **Which kind of muscle controls the blood vessels?**

Smooth.

○   **Which kind of muscle is found in the urinary and intestinal tracts?**

Smooth.

○   **Which kind of muscle possesses the quality of automaticity?**

Cardiac.

○   **In what way are cardiac and smooth muscle similar?**

They are both involuntary.

MYOCARDIAL INFARCTION AND STROKE

❍ **What is the most common cause of out-of-hospital cardiac arrest?**

Ventricular fibrillation. Other causes include ventricular tachycardia, supraventricular tachydysrhythmias, and bradydysrhythmias.

❍ **What are the signs and symptoms of congestive heart failure?**

Shortness of breath, tachypnea, cyanosis, labored respirations, jugular venous distention, S3 gallop.

❍ **What is a transmural myocardial infarction?**

An infarction involving the entire thickness of the myocardium. It is also called a Q-wave infarction.

❍ **What is a subendocardial infarction?**

An infarction is limited to the subendocardial layer of the myocardium. It is also called a non-Q-wave infarction.

❍ **Why is it important to relieve the pain of a myocardial infarction?**

Decreases oxygen demand, dysrhythmias, blood pressure and heart rate, and relieves anxiety.

❍ **What are the criteria of treating a myocardial infarction with thrombolytic therapy?**

- Chest pain lasting longer than 20 minutes.
- S-T segment elevation equal to or greater than 1 mm in two or more contiguous leads (2, 3, AVF; 1 and AVL; V1-V6).
- Patient seen within six hours of symptom onset.
- No absolute contraindications to thrombolytic therapy.

❍ **What is the danger of hypertension in a patient with myocardial infarction?**

Risk of increasing myocardial oxygen demand, myocardial ischemia, and exacerbating infarction.

O   **After symptom onset, when is the greatest risk of death from a myocardial infarction?**

Within two hours.

O   **What are the goals of thrombolytic therapy?**

Restoration of blood flow through the infarct related artery, thus improving myocardial oxygenation, decreasing myocardial ischemia, improving left ventricular function and cardiac output, improving arterial perfusion, decreasing dysrhythmias, and reducing mortality.

O   **What is afterload?**

Resistance against which the heart pumps to eject blood. This is usually measured by the systemic blood pressure.

O   **What is pulseless electrical activity?**

When a spontaneous rhythm is seen on the monitor but no detectable pulse is palpable.

O   **What are the key features of unstable angina?**

Angina at rest, new onset angina, angina induced by minimal exertion, and an increase of severity, frequency or duration of anginal attacks.

O   **What is the effect of nitroglycerin in the treatment of acute pulmonary edema?**

Nitroglycerin increases venous capacitance and reduces preload and afterload.

O   **What is preload?**

Preload is the filling pressure of the left ventricle before systolic contraction.

O   **What is the effect of parasympathetic nerve fiber stimulation on the heart?**

Acetylcholine release resulting in a decreased rate of discharge in the sinus node, decreased conduction through the A-V node, and a decrease in heart rate.

O   **What are the signs and symptoms of right heart failure?**

Diaphoresis, tachycardia, dyspnea, jugular venous distention, dependent edema, and fatigue.

❍　**What are the common signs and symptoms of cardiogenic shock?**

Cool clammy skin, hypotension, tachycardia, tachypnea, restlessness, confusion, depressed mental status, and signs and symptoms of myocardial infarction.

❍　**What are the common causes of cardiac arrest?**

Ventricular fibrillation due to myocardial infarction is the most common. Other causes include drowning, hypoxia, electrocution, drug overdose, hypothermia, acid-base imbalance, electrolyte imbalance, and trauma.

❍　**What is the most common cause of anterior or lateral wall infarctions?**

Occlusion of a branch of the left coronary artery.

❍　**What is the ECG hallmark of non-Q-wave infarcts?**

When an abnormal level of cardiac serum markers, such as troponin or CPK are released, but only S-T segment deviation or T-wave abnormalities occur.

❍　**T/F: Patients with non-Q-wave infarcts have a lower in-hospital mortality rate than patients with Q wave infarcts.**

True. However, they also have a higher incidence of long-term cardiac events, such as recurrent ischemia, reinfarction and death.

❍　**T/F: Most episodes of acute coronary syndrome occur at rest or modest daily activity.**

True. Heavy physical exertion or stress is only present in a small minority of patients.

❍　**What is the most common time of day to suffer from an acute myocardial infarction?**

Between 6:00 a.m. and 10:00 a.m. The second most common time is in the early evening.

❍　**What is the most common symptom of acute myocardial infarction?**

Substernal chest pain.

❍　**In the first few hours following a myocardial infarction, what is the most common complication?**

Ventricular and/or atrial dysrhythmias.

○ **An 85 year-old presents with diffuse rales and shortness of breath. Blood pressure is 60/40, respiratory rate is 30, and the heart rate is 120 beats per minute. Chest x-ray reveals florid pulmonary edema. What is the treatment?**

IV, O2, and monitor and a dopamine drip starting at 10 mcg/kg/min titrated to a maximum of 20 mcg/kg/min or until the systolic blood pressure is at least 90 mmHg.

○ **What is the most common cause of cardiogenic shock?**

It is most often due to extensive myocardial infarction, typically involving 40% or more of the left ventricle.

○ **What is the most common cause of inferior wall myocardial infarction?**

Right coronary artery occlusion.

○ **What are the clinical findings in pericardial tamponade?**

Distended neck veins, muffled heart sounds, narrowing pulse pressure, hypotension, and pulseless paradoxus.

○ **You are managing a patient in acute cardiac arrest. From the monitor, you cannot tell if the rhythm is fine ventricular fibrillation or asystole. What is the initial treatment?**

Assume the patient has ventricular fibrillation and defibrillate the patient.

○ **What type of dysrhythmias are associated with inferior wall MIs?**

First degree A-V block, second degree A-V block, Mobitz Type I, third degree A-V block with junctional escape rhythm, ventricular fibrillation and sinus bradycardia.

○ **What are some of the most common metabolic causes of cardiac arrest?**

Hypokalemia and antidysrhythmic drug treatment. Other causes include hypomagnesemia and toxic reactions to drugs such as cocaine, tricyclic antidepressants, and phenothiazines.

○ **What findings are evident on an ECG in a patient suffering a myocardial infarction?**

S-T segment elevation and T-wave inversion. Long term Q-waves may be apparent due to the lack of depolarization of infarcted tissue.

❍ **What is the effect of calcium channel blockers?**

Decreased myocardial oxygen demand, relaxation of vascular smooth muscle, and dilatation of the coronary arteries.

❍ **What are the main branches of the right coronary artery?**

The posterior descending artery and the marginal artery.

❍ **What are the main branches of the left coronary artery?**

Anterior descending artery and circumflex artery.

❍ **What are the signs and symptoms of stroke?**

Weakness, dyscoordination, facial weakness and asymmetry, incoherent speech, inability to speak (aphasia), ataxia, visual disturbances, confusion or altered level of consciousness, coma, hearing loss, vertigo, nausea, vomiting, headache, and photophobia.

❍ **What is an ischemic stroke?**

When an artery is blocked by a thrombus or a blood clot which is developed in a peripheral source such as the heart or blood vessels and travels to the brain resulting in an embolic event.

❍ **What is a hemorrhagic stroke?**

Hemorrhagic stroke is a result of a ruptured blood vessel.

❍ **What are the immediate treatments of a patient who has suffered increased intracranial pressure as the result of a suspected stroke?**

Elevate the head of the bed, fluid restriction, intubate and hyperventilate, control pain and agitation, and treat with mannitol 1-2 g/kg IV. The patient should be hyperventilated to a PCO2 of 25-28 mmHg.

❍ **What fluid rate should be used in a stroke victim?**

Fluid should be administered at a very slow rate unless the patient is hypotensive.

❍ **Does a normal ECG tracing rule out a myocardial infarction?**

No.

○ **Why is aspirin used in the treatment of acute myocardial infarction?**

Blocks clotting by inhibiting prostaglandin synthesis of platelets, thereby inhibiting platelet aggregation.

○ **While monitoring a patient admitted to the coronary care unit with an acute myocardial infarction, you notice the onset of multiform ventricular extra-systoles that rapidly progresses to ventricular fibrillation. Your assessment reveals a pulseless, apneic patient. Your next therapy should be:**

a. a precordial thump
b. closed chest compressions
c. endotracheal intubation
d. lidocaine 1 mg/kg IV bolus
e. immediate defibrillation with 200 J

Answer: **E**

○ **Cardiac compromise is often a problem associated with the pre-hospital setting. List several signs and symptoms of a patient who may be suffering cardiac compromise.**

A squeezing feeling in the chest, dull pressure, chest pain commonly radiating down the arms or into the jaw, a sudden onset of sweating. There can be difficulty in breathing, anxiety, irritability, a feeling of impending doom, abnormal pulse rate that may be irregular, abnormal blood pressure, epigastric pain, nausea, and vomiting.

○ **Describe the appropriate emergency medical care for a patient who is complaining of having chest discomfort with related heart disease.**

Assess baseline vital signs. Administer oxygen. Encourage patient to cease all activity. Have him sit in a position of comfort. Loosen tight clothing around waist and neck. Begin obtaining a focused assessment.

○ **Identify several things the rescuer should question the patient about their chest discomfort.**

When did the pain start? What caused the pain to begin? Have the patient rate the quality of the pain, 1 being the lowest and 10 being the worst pain he has have ever experienced. Is there any radiation of the pain to the arm, neck, or jaw? Is there any associated shortness of breath? Is there any increased intensity of the discomfort with breathing or change in posture?

○   **Describe the proper procedure for administering nitroglycerin to a patient complaining of chest pain.**

Determine if nitroglycerin has been prescribed to the patient and if it is with the patient. Assess the patient's blood pressure to ensure that the systolic pressure is higher than 100 mmHg. You may administer one dose and repeat in 3-5 minutes if no relief and authorized by medical direction, up to a maximum of three doses. Reassess vital signs and chest discomfort after each dose. If the patient's blood pressure is less than 100 mmHg systolic, continue with the elements of the focused assessment and do not administer the nitroglycerin.

○   **Describe the treatment of a patient complaining of chest discomfort who does not have prescribed nitroglycerin.**

A patient who does not have prescribed nitroglycerin should be given oxygen at 15L/min via non-rebreather mask while continuing with the focused assessment. Transport promptly. Assess the need for advanced life support.

○   **Identify the proper procedure for administering a nitroglycerin tablet to a patient with chest pain.**

Obtain order from medical direction either on-line or off-line. Perform a focused cardiac assessment. Assess the blood pressure to ensure a systolic of greater than 100 mmHg. Contact medical control if there are no standing orders. Ensure that you have the right medication, the right patient, the right route, and the patient is alert and up to taking the product. Check the expiration date of the nitroglycerin. Question the patient as to last dose, the effects, and ensure that he understands the he is going to take his own medication. Ask the patient to lift his tongue and place the tablet or spray dose under the tongue while wearing protective gloves. Have the patient keep his mouth closed with the tablet under the tongue without swallowing until it is dissolved and absorbed. Recheck the blood pressure within two minutes. Have the patient rest. Provide high flow oxygen via non-rebreather mask. Prepare for transfer to the local hospital.

○   **Describe the actions of nitroglycerin upon the patient after taking the medication.**

Decreased the workload of the heart and dilation of blood vessels, which allows for greater blood flow to the heart muscle.

○   **Identify the reassessment strategies an you should use when administering nitroglycerin to a cardiac patient.**

Monitor the blood pressure every 3-5 minutes. Ask the patient about effect on pain relief. Seek medical direction before administering a second dosage and record all reassessments.

POST-TEST

○   **Which of the following rhythms is most commonly present in the first minute following a cardiac arrest in adults?**

a. ventricular tachycardia
b. asystole
c. bradycardia
d. ventricular fibrillation

Answer: **D**

○   **What is the drug treatment priority list in treating unstable bradycardia?**

Oxygen, then atropine, then a dopamine drip at 5-20 mcg/kg/min then epinephrine at 2-10 mcg/min.

○   **Drugs useful in the treatment of cardiogenic pulmonary edema include:**

a. furosemide
b. verapamil
c. morphine
d. propanolol
e. oxygen

Answer: **A, C and E.**

○   **An 80 year-old presents with severe chest pain. Heart rate is 30 and blood pressure is 60/P mmHg. The monitor shows sinus bradycardia. Which drug is indicated first?**

a. lidocaine 75 mg IV bolus
b. isoproterenol infusion at 2 - 10 mcg/min
c. atropine 0.5-1 mg IV
d. morphine 2 - 5 mg IV

Answer: **C**

○   **Intubation with an endotracheal tube:**

a. allows adjunctive ventilatory equipment to be used effectively
b. decreases the risk of aspiration

c. is the first priority in ventricular fibrillation
d. performed improperly may result in only one lung being inflated

Answer: **A, B, and D**

O   **Bag-valve-mask devices:**

a. may be used by untrained individuals
b. with high flow and a reservoir deliver close to 100% oxygen
c. are difficult for one person to use effectively
d. usually provide greater tidal volume than mouth-to-mask ventilation

Answer: **B and C**

O   **During cardiac arrest, acidosis:**

a. usually is both metabolic and respiratory
b. should be treated with increased ventilation
c. should generally be treated with sodium bicarbonate
d. usually resolves once perfusion is restored

Answer: **A, B, and D**

O   **Which of the following is true in regards to endotracheal suction?**

a. Limited to 15 seconds
b. Preceded with oxygen ventilation
c. Can result in hypoxia
d. Perform without applying suction

Answer: **All of the above**

O   **After placement of an endotracheal tube, ventilate:**

a. at 10 - 15 breaths per minute
b. after the 5th compression
c. asynchronously to cardiac compressions
d. with room air

Answer: **A and C**

O   **Breath sounds cannot be heard following endotracheal intubation. What is the most likely problem?**

Answer: **Esophageal intubation**

○ **Which of the following patients require intubation?**

a. conscious with a suspected stroke
b. unconscious with no gag reflex
c. normotensive with third degree heart block
d. cardiac arrest after 3 unsuccessful countershocks

Answer: **B and D**

○ **Endotracheal intubation complications include:**

Vocal cord injury, dental damage, esophageal intubation, and right main bronchus intubation

○ **In a patient refractory to atropine, when is external pacing indicated?**

a. pulseless electrical activity
b. agonal rhythm
c. symptomatic bradycardia
d. symptomatic ventricular fibrillation

Answer: **C**

○ **You have been unsuccessful in the first two attempts to defibrillate an adult. The energy for the third defibrillation attempt is:**

a. 50 J
b. 100 J
c. 200 - 300 J
d. 360 J

Answer: **D**

○ **Greater defibrillating current is expected with which of the following?**

a. successive countershocks
b. firm paddle pressure
c. use of conductive medium
d. lower body weight

Answer: **A, B, and C**

○ **For a deeply unconscious patient in shock, what is the airway of choice?**

a. endotracheal tube
b. esophageal obturator

c. oropharyngeal
d. nasopharyngeal

Answer: **D**

○   **In an unconscious or semi-conscious patient an oropharyngeal airway:**

a. eliminates the need for head positioning
b. eliminates upper airway obstruction
c. has no value once an endotracheal tube is inserted
d. may stimulate vomiting or laryngospasm

Answer: **D**

○   **CPR is in progress. Immediately upon diagnosing the following rhythm, what is the treatment?**

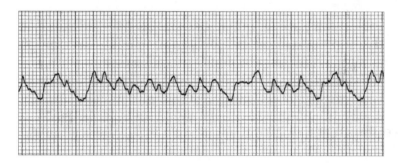

a. administer lidocaine
b. precordial thump
c. synchronized shock with 200 J
d. unsynchronized shock with 200 J

Answer: **D** (The above rhythm shows ventricular fibrillation).

○   **Atropine may:**

a. not be given via the endotracheal tube
b. exacerbate ischemia in an acute MI
c. cause tachycardia
d. increase the rate of sinus bradycardia

Answer: **B, C, and D**

○   **The recommended dose of epinephrine injected into the adult tracheobronchial tree should be:**

2.0 - 2.5 times the IV dose in 10 ml of solution

○ **Nitroglycerin:**

a. may be given sublingually or IV
b. is useful in relieving chest pain in acute myocardial infarction
c. causes hypotension
d. may be repeated more than once

Answer: **All of the above**

○ **Dopamine infused at greater than 10 mcg/kg/min will cause:**

a. increased myocardial contractility
b. peripheral arterial vasoconstriction
c. renal artery vasoconstriction
d. respiratory depression

Answer: **A, B and C**

○ **Dopamine at low doses (1 - 2 mcg/kg/min) will cause:**

a. elevated blood pressure
b. renal vasoconstriction
c. renal vasodilatation
d. tachycardia

Answer: **C**

○ **Sodium bicarbonate should be considered in arrests caused by:**

Tricyclic overdose, hyperkalemia, and pre-existing metabolic acidosis

○ **In the treatment of an 80-kg adult in ventricular tachycardia with a pulse, which of the following schedules of lidocaine is preferred?**

a. 80 mg IV bolus followed by an infusion at 2 - 4 mg/min
b. 160 mg IV bolus every 10 minutes up to a total of 500 mg
c. 160 mg IV bolus followed by an infusion at 6 mg/min
d. 400 mg IV bolus followed by an infusion at 1 - 2 mg/min

Answer: **A**

○ **T/F: Bradycardia not responding to atropine should be treated with isoproterenol 1 mg in 250 ml D5W infused wide open.**

False.

○   **T/F: Lidocaine enhances myocardial contractility.**

False.

○   **T/F: Beta-blockers depress the pumping function of heart muscle.**

True.

○   **Describe the use of a curved versus straight laryngoscope blade.**

The curved blade is designed to fit into the vallecula whereas the straight blade is used to lift the epiglottis.

○   **What cardiac drugs should be avoided in acute cardiogenic pulmonary edema?**

Beta-blockers, such as propranolol, and isoproterenol.

○   **T/F: Antishock garments should be used to treat acute cardiogenic pulmonary edema.**

False.

○   **T/F: Ventricular fibrillation produces no cardiac output.**

True.

○   **What is the effect of atropine on vagal reflexes?**

Atropine typically decreases vagal reflexes while increasing ventricular irritability.

○   **Regarding epinephrine, which of the following statements are true?**

a. increases coronary perfusion
b. IV bolus dose is 1 mg q 3-5 minutes
c. treatment for hypotensive ventricular tachycardia
d. increases cerebral blood flow during CPR

Answer: **A, B, and C**

○   **What are the end points of a procainamide loading infusion in the non-arrest situation?**

a. pre-treatment QRS complex is widened by 50%
b. hypotension
c. 17 mg/kg drug has been injected
d. the dysrhythmia is suppressed

Answer: **All of the above**

○   **A patient is in ventricular fibrillation that has failed to respond to several defibrillations or lidocaine. What is the treatment?**

Following the secondary survey for airway management and CPR, amiodarone 300 mg IVP, followed by 150 mg IVP every 3-5 minutes up to a maximum dose of 2.2 grams IV per 24 hours. Procainamide 50 mg/min IV infusion (urgent situation) up to total dose of 17 mg/kg and/or Magnesium sulfate IVP can be given. Bretylium use is no longer recommended.

○   **Why use an endotracheal tube stylet?**

To make the tube form fitting.

○   **What type of drug is verapamil?**

Calcium channel blocker.

○   **What type of drug is propranolol?**

A beta-blocker.

○   **What is the mechanism of action of adenosine on the heart?**

Depresses sinus node and A-V node activity.

○   **T/F: A pop-off valve is desirable when selecting a bag-valve-mask device.**

False. Desirable features include: transparent mask, non-rebreathing valve, and a self-expanding bag.

○   **In what type of rhythm may lidocaine be lethal?**

Idioventricular rhythm or complete heart block.

○   **T/F: Infectious complications of intravenous cannulas should be prevented by using systemic antibiotics.**

False.

○   **What is the appropriate dose of a medication given by endotracheal tube?**

Two to two-and-a-half times the IV dose.

○   **T/F: Verapamil should be used when the origin of a wide complex tachycardia**

is unknown.

False.

○   **A 60 year-old presents with a blood pressure of 80/40, heart rate is 200, and respiratory rate is 24. The nurse has placed oxygen on the patient. The following rhythm is seen on the monitor. What is the treatment?**

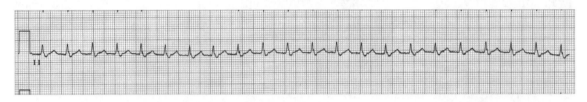

Synchronized cardioversion.   (The rhythm seen above shows supraventricular tachycardia).

○   **In therapeutic doses, which drug depresses the pumping function of the heart muscle?**

a. atropine
b. epinephrine
c. propanolol
d. isoproterenol

Answer: **C.**

○   **Calcium chloride should be considered in an overdose of:**

a. bretylium
b. epinephrine
c. verapamil
d. procainamide

Answer: **C**

○   **Infectious complications of intravenous cannulas can be decreased by:**

Using aseptic technique during insertion, replacing the cannula after 3 days, and keeping the stopcock on when not in use.   Prophylactic antibiotics are not indicated in most patients.

○   **Complications of transcutaneous pacing include:**

Delay in recognizing VF, failure to capture, and skin burns.   There is no risk of electric shock to the operator.

❍   **A common lethal complication of lightning strike is:**

a. stroke
b. cardiac tamponade
c. congestive heart failure
d. respiratory arrest

Answer: **D**

❍   **In rescuing a near drowning victim, the rescuer should:**

a. compress the chest to drain water from breathing passages
b. assure their own safety
c. stabilize the cervical spine if a diving accident
d. start rescue breathing

Answer: **B, C, and D**

❍   **Expansion of circulating fluid volume with normal saline is recommended in all cardiac arrests.**

False.

❍   **The preferred vein for initial cannulation during CPR is the:**

a. external jugular vein
b. femoral vein
c. subclavian vein
d. antecubital vein

Answer: **D**

❍   **AC shock tends to cause?**

a. asystole
b. respiratory arrest
c. bradycardia
d. ventricular fibrillation

Answer: **D**

❍   **Traumatic injuries may include all of the following except:**

a. cardiac tamponade
b. hyperkalemia
c. shock

d. tension pneumothorax

Answer: **B**

○   **After initiating CPR, which one of the following treatments should be used for treating ventricular fibrillation?**

a. intubation
b. defibrillation
c. epinephrine IV
d. lidocaine IV

Answer: **B**

○   **A patient has the following rhythm refractory to adenosine IV and verapamil IV. Before treatment, the heart rate was 200 beats/min and his blood pressure was 110/70 mmHg. After treatment, the heart rate remains at 200 beats/minute and the blood pressure is 60 mmHg systolic. What should the immediate treatment be?**

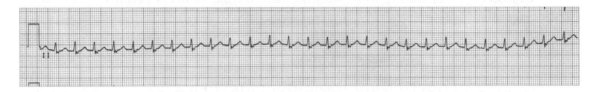

a. atropine 0.5 mg IV
b. dopamine drip IV
c. synchronized cardioversion at 50 - 100 J
d. verapamil 10 mg IV over 1 - 2 minutes

Answer: **C.** (The rhythm above shows supraventricular tachycardia).

○   **A 40 year-old presents pale and diaphoretic. The heart rate is 200 beats per minute and blood pressure is 60 mmHg palpable. The monitor reveals the following rhythm. Oxygen is applied. What is the recommended immediate treatment?**

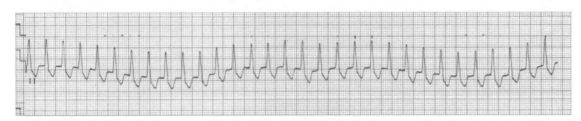

a. procainamide
b. propanolol
c. synchronized cardioversion at 50 - 100 J
d. verapamil

Answer: **C.** (The above rhythm shows supraventricular tachycardia).

○ **A 60 year-old complains of chest pain for 60 minutes. The patient is cool and clammy, heart rate is 40 beats/min, and blood pressure is 70/50 mmHg. The monitor shows the following rhythm. What is the recommended immediate treatment?**

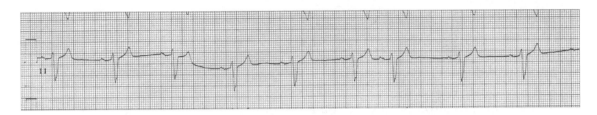

a. atropine 0.5-1 mg IV push
b. dopamine IV infusion 20 mcg/kg/min
c. epinephrine 1 mg IV push
d. transcutaneous pacemaker

Answer: **A.** (The rhythm shown above is sinus bradycardia).

○ **You are performing synchronized cardioversion when the following rhythm suddenly appears. What is the recommended immediate treatment?**

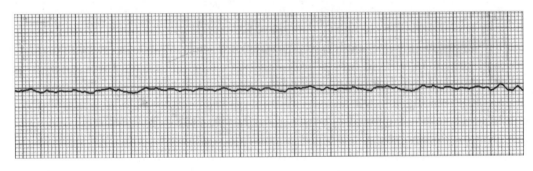

a. lidocaine 100 mg IV bolus
b. begin CPR
c. unsynchronized countershock at 200 J
d. synchronized shock at 200 J

Answer: **C.** (The above rhythm is ventricular fibrillation).

○ **A patient with a myocardial infarction develops the following rhythm and loses consciousness. The patient is pulseless and not breathing. What is the preferred immediate treatment?**

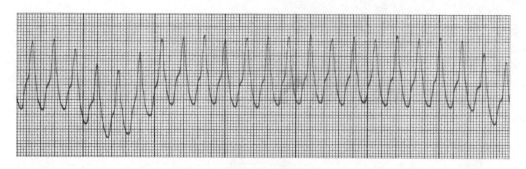

a. administer bretylium
b. administer lidocaine
c. call for help and deliver a synchronized shock
d. call for help and deliver an unsynchronized shock

Answer: **D.** (The above rhythm shows ventricular tachycardia).

❍   **Paramedics arrive at the scene and find an unresponsive patient. EMTs have already established an IV and CPR is in progress. There is no pulse. The monitor shows the following rhythm. What should the paramedics do?**

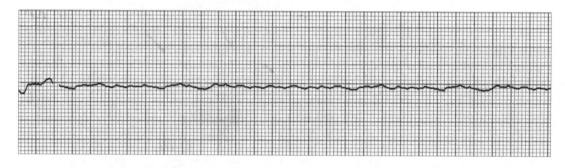

a. immediate defibrillation followed by setup of the automatic external defibrillator.
b. administer epinephrine, 1 ml of 1:10,000 solution
c. administer epinephrine, 10 ml of 1:10,000 solution, then defibrillate
d. administer sodium bicarbonate 50 mEq IV bolus

Answer: **A.** (The above rhythm shows fine ventricular fibrillation).

❍   **T/F: Mouth-to-mask ventilation usually provides greater tidal volume than bag-valve-mask devices.**

True.

❍   **Should suction be applied while performing endotracheal suction?**

No. Avoid suction while inserting the catheter.

○   When giving a patient epinephrine via the endotracheal tube, the proper dose should be 2-2.5 times the recommended IV dose. How much normal saline should be used?

10 ml of normal saline.

○   When should sodium bicarbonate be considered in cardiac arrest?

In hyperkalemia, in patients with known metabolic acidosis, and in tricyclic antidepressant overdose. It should not be given in hypoxic lactic acidosis.

○   T/F: Epinephrine increases cerebral and myocardial blood flow during CPR.

True.

○   T/F: Epinephrine increases coronary perfusion pressure.

True.

○   T/F: Propranolol increases the pumping function of heart muscle.

False.   Beta-blockers depress contractility.

○   While working in the CCU taking care of a patient with a myocardial infarction, you notice the sudden onset of ventricular fibrillation.   Further evaluation reveals a pulseless patient. What should you do next?

CPR and shock therapy as soon as possible.

○   A patient complains of shortness of breath and chest pain radiating to the neck. Blood pressure is 80/50 mmHg and the respiratory rate is 40 per minute. Oxygen and an IV has been started.   The monitor shows the following rhythm. What should the next treatment be?

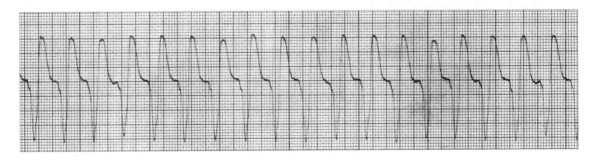

a. carotid massage
b. lidocaine
c. sedation, then synchronized cardioversion

d. adenosine

Answer: **C.** (The above rhythm is a wide-complex QRS tachycardia, rate 160/minute).

○   **A 70-kg emergency department patient has pulseless electrical activity. An IV is started and a saline infusion is begun. What should the first treatment be?**

a. lidocaine 70 mg
b. epinephrine 1 mg IV
c. verapamil 5 mg IV
d. sodium bicarbonate 1 ampule

Answer: **B**

○   **What is the evaluation and treatment for a patient with pulseless electrical activity?**

CPR, rapid fluid challenge, Oxygen, check breath sounds bilaterally and give epinephrine.

○   **The three most treatable causes of pulseless electrical activity are:**

a. massive pulmonary embolism
b. cardiac tamponade
c. hypovolemia
d. tension pneumothorax
e. massive myocardial infarction

Answer: **B, C, and D**

○   **Ventricular fibrillation:**

a. may be mimicked by artifact on the monitor
b. may produce a peripheral pulse
c. produces no cardiac output
d. treated with early defibrillation

Answer: **A, C, and D**

○   **Following successful resuscitation from ventricular fibrillation, patients should be treated with:**

Oxygen and lidocaine.

○ During cardiac arrest from pulseless electrical activity, the exam reveals distended neck veins. How should cardiac tamponade be ruled out?

Pericardiocentesis.

○ A patient with the following rhythm is successfully shocked into a sinus rhythm with a pulse. What is the recommended initial treatment?

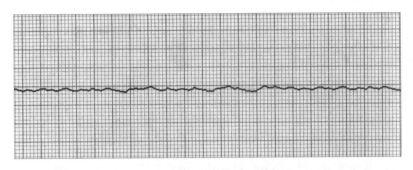

Oxygen and intravenous lidocaine 1.0 mg/kg/bolus, followed by an infusion of 2-4 mg/min. (The rhythm above shows fine ventricular fibrillation).

○ An intubated patient develops sudden onset narrow complex tachycardia, at a rate of 130 beats per minute. Vital signs are 0-0-0. CPR is in progress. The most important action is:

a. Find the cause of the arrest
b. Give 1 mg epinephrine IVP
c. Give verapamil 5 mg IVP
d. Cardiovert at 360 J

Answer: **B**

○ A patient's heart rate is 40 beats/min with a systolic blood pressure of 50 mmHg. A transcutaneous pacemaker is not available. List the treatments in order of priority:

Oxygenation, atropine, dopamine, epinephrine

○ Which of the following drugs are not used in the routine management of an acute MI?

a. lidocaine
b. oxygen
c. nitroglycerin
d. morphine

Answer: **A**

○   **If no contraindications exist, thrombolytic therapy should be given to patients with:**

a. chest pain for 4 hours with clear ST elevation > 1mm in two adjacent leads
b. presentation within 12 hours after symptom onset
c. 6 hours of chest pain and left bundle branch block
d. 6 hours of chest pain, ST elevation, and age greater than 75 years

Answer: **A, C, and D**

○   **Potentially treatable causes of asystole include:**

Hypoxia, acidosis, hyperkalemia and tension pneumothorax.

○   **A 5 year-old child is evaluated by paramedics for "difficulty breathing". Paramedics find the child is not breathing, is pulseless and apneic. The monitor shows a bradyarrhythmia at 30 beats/min. What should be the first intervention?**

Check the airway.

○   **Transcutaneous cardiac pacing is appropriate for the following situations:**

a. sinus bradycardia
b. sinus bradycardia with hypotension
c. complete heart block with pulmonary edema
d. prolonged asystole

Answer: **A and B**

○   **T/F: Brain damage, after resuscitation, is evidence of negligence:**

False.

○   **T/F: An automated defibrillator can accurately diagnose ventricular fibrillation during chest compressions.**

False.

○   **An Advanced Cardiac Life Support card, implies:**

a. Expertise in ACLS according to the guidelines of the American Heart Association
b. Certification to prescribe the treatments taught in the ACLS course
c. Qualification to perform the procedures taught in ACLS in a hospital setting
d. Successful completion of a course in ACLS according to the guidelines of the American Heart Association and the Heart and Stroke Foundation of Canada

Answer: **D**

○ **A patient is apneic and pulseless. The following is the presenting rhythm. Treatment?**

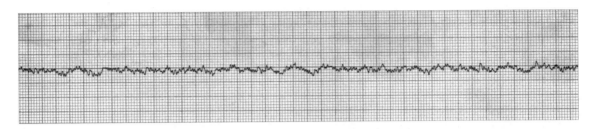

Defibrillate with 200 J, 200-300 J, then 360 J (checking pulse and rhythm after each defibrillation), intubate, IV access. If spontaneous rhythm and pulse are not restored, begin CPR and give epinephrine 1 mg IV push. (The rhythm above shows ventricular fibrillation).

○ **The patient is pulseless and apneic with the following rhythm. Bag-mask ventilations and chest compressions are begun. Treatment?**

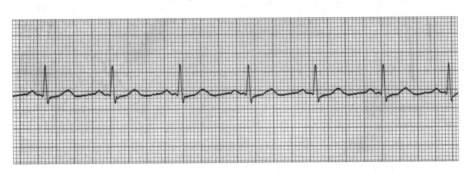

CPR, intubate and administer epinephrine. (The rhythm above reveals pulseless electrical activity or PEA).

○ **A 44 year-old patient is admitted to hospital with community-acquired pneumonia and started on IV erythromycin. Suddenly, he is found unresponsive on the floor. A code is called, and, transiently, the patient's rhythm is seen below. What is the rhythm and what is the treatment?**

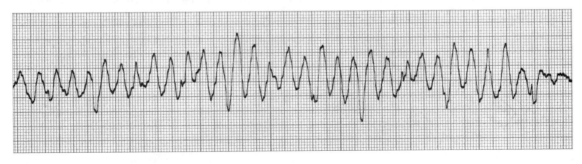

The rhythm is Torsades de Pointes, a form of ventricular tachycardia. This rhythm is most often transient, due to prolongation of the Q-T interval. The recommended treatment is to discontinue erythromycin, a well-known, but uncommon cause of Torsades de Pointes. More common causes include Quinidine, Procainamde, Flecainide, tricyclic antidepressants, Phenothiazines.

❍ **A patient complains of nausea, weakness, and shortness of breath. The patient is cool and clammy. BP 70/50, pulse 30, respirations 28. The monitor shows the following rhythm. Order of treatment?**

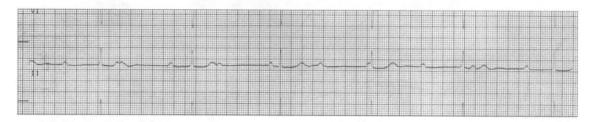

O_2, atropine, pacemaker, dopamine, epinephrine, isoproterenol. (The rhythm above is 3° AV block).

❍ **An 80 year-old complains of chest pain that began one hour ago. The patient is pale and diaphoretic. BP is 80/50, respiratory rate is 24. The monitor shows the following rhythm. Treatment?**

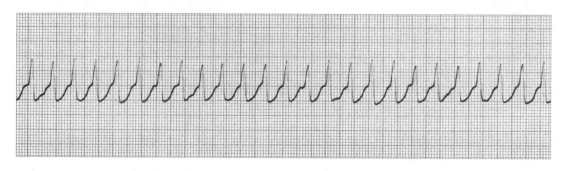

Consider sedation and synchronized countershock with 100 J. (The rhythm above is ventricular tachycardia).

❍ **A patient in the CCU complains of sudden dizziness, nausea, vomiting, and difficulty breathing. Exam reveals rales throughout both lung fields, BP is 80/50, and respirations are 40/min. The monitor shows the following rhythm. Treatment?**

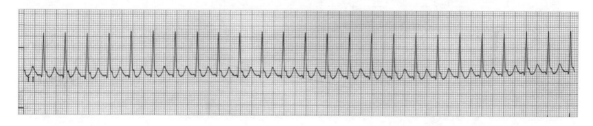

IV access, O_2, monitor, IV sedation followed by synchronized cardioversion at 100 J.

(The rhythm above shows paroxysmal supraventricular tachycardia).

O **The patient has been in the following rhythm for 2 - 3 minutes. Treatment?**

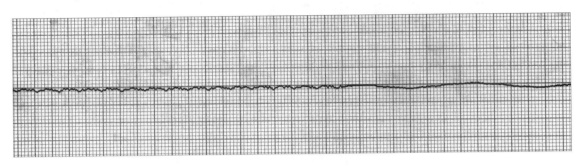

CPR, epinephrine, atropine, consider transcutaneous pacemaker. (The rhythm above shows asystole).

O **The patient "fainted". Exam reveals an alert patient. BP is 120/80 and respirations are 16/min. The patient denies chest pain or injuries. The monitor shows the following rhythm. Treatment?**

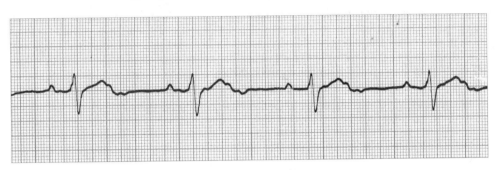

O_2, IV access, transcutaneous pacer on standby, monitor closely and rapid transport to a facility for likely permanent pacemaker implantation. (The rhythm above is 2° AV block, Mobitz Type II).

O **Describe the function of the right atrium of the heart.**

The right atrium receives blood from the large veins in the body and pumps oxygen- poor blood to the right ventricle.

O **Describe the function of the left atrium.**

The left atrium receives blood from the pulmonary veins located in the lungs and pumps oxygenated blood to the left ventricle.

O **Inadequate tissue perfusion is the definition of what?**

Shock.

○ **Describe the proper technique for assessing circulation in infants and children.**

When assessing the circulatory status of a child, the following need to be examined; the brachial or femoral pulse, peripheral pulses, capillary refill, skin color and temperature. Blood pressure should be assessed in children over the age of 3.

○ **Describe the function of the right ventricle.**

The right ventricle pumps blood to the lungs to be oxygenated.

○ **Describe the function of the left ventricle.**

The left ventricle pumps blood to the rest of the body.

○ **Describe the function of the valves located within the heart.**

The valves located within the heart prevent back-flow of blood into the chambers from which it came.

○ **Describe a unique characteristic of the heart muscle itself that is not found in any other muscle in the body.**

Cardiac muscle is unique in that it contains its own conductive system.

○ **Describe the function of the arteries that are located within the body.**

Arteries carry blood from the heart to the rest of the body.

○ **What is the function of the coronary arteries?**

To supply blood to the heart muscle.

○ **Describe the major function of the aorta.**

The aorta is the major artery originating from the heart and lying in front of the spine in the thoracic and abdominal cavities. This provides blood flow to the rest of the vascular system in the body.

○ **Describe the location and function of the pulmonary artery.**

The pulmonary artery originates in the right ventricle. Its function is to carry oxygen poor blood to the lungs.

○   **Describe the location and function of the carotid artery.**

The carotid artery is located in the neck. It supplies the head with blood. Pulsation can be palpated on either side of the neck.

○   **Describe the location and function of the femoral artery.**

The femoral artery is the major artery of the thigh. It supplies the groin and lower extremities with blood. Pulsation can be palpated in the groin.

○   **Describe the location of the radial artery.**

The radial artery is the artery that provides blood supply to the lower hand. Pulsation can be palpated at the wrists on the thumb side.

○   **Describe the location and function of the brachial artery.**

The brachial artery is found in the upper arm and supplies blood to the humerus, the biceps, and triceps. Pulsation can be palpated on the inside of the arm between the elbow and shoulder. The brachial artery is often used when measuring a blood pressure with a blood pressure cuff and a stethoscope.

○   **Describe where you would find the posterior tibial pulse.**

On the posterior surface of the medial malleolus.

○   **Identify the location of arterioles within the circulatory system.**

Arterioles are the smallest branches of an artery leading to the capillaries.

○   **Describe the location and function of capillaries.**

Capillaries are tiny blood vessels that connect arterioles to venules. They are found in all parts of the body. Their function is to allow the exchange of nutrients and waste at the cellular level.

○   **What are venules?**

Venules are the smallest branches of veins leading to the capillaries.

○   **Identify the function of veins within the cardiovascular system.**

Veins are vessels that carry de-oxygenated blood back to the heart. The only exception to this is the pulmonary veins, which carry oxygenated blood from the lungs back to the heart.

○   **What is the function of the pulmonary vein?**

To carry oxygen rich blood from the lungs to the left atrium for distribution to the rest of the body.

○   **What is the location and function of the vena cava?**

The vena cava is broken into two sections, the superior vena cava, which originates in the upper chest, and the inferior vena cava, which originates in the abdomen. The function of the vena cava is to carry this blood to the right atrium.

○   **What is the function of red blood cells?**

To carry oxygen to the organs of the body and to carry carbon dioxide away from those organs.

○   **What is the function of white blood cells within the circulatory system?**

White blood cells act as part of the body's defense against infection.

○   **Describe the function of plasma as it relates to the circulatory system.**

Plasma is the fluid that carries the blood cells and nutrients.

○   **Describe the function of platelets within the cardiovascular system.**

Platelets are essential for the formation of blood clots.

○   **Describe the meaning of the term pulse as it relates to the cardiovascular system and explain where a pulse could be palpated.**

The pulse is what is felt when the left ventricle contracts and sends a wave of blood through the arteries. It can be palpated anywhere an artery simultaneously passes near the skin's surface.

○   **Identify four primary sites where a peripheral pulse may be palpated.**

Radial, brachial, posterior tibial, and dorsalis pedis.

○   **Identify two areas in which a central pulse may be palpated.**

The carotid artery in the neck or the femoral artery in the groin.

❍ **What is meant by the following two terms as they relate to blood pressure: systolic and diastolic.**

Systolic is the pressure exerted against the walls of the artery when the left ventricle contracts. Diastolic is the pressure exerted against the walls of the artery when the left ventricle is at rest.

❍ **Shock is also called hypoperfusion. Identify the meaning of inadequate circulation as it relates to shock.**

Shock or inadequate circulation is a state of profound depression of the vital processes of the body. It is characterized by signs and symptoms such as palor; cyanosis; cool, clammy skin; rapid, weak pulse; rapid, shallow breathing; restlessness, anxiety, or mental dullness; nausea and vomiting; reduction in the total blood volume; and hypotension.

❍ **Identify five ways in which a patient may lose heat.**

Radiation, convection, conduction, evaporation, breathing.

❍ **Identify the condition in which a patient's heat loss exceeds the patient's heat gain.**

Hypothermia.

❍ **Identify the condition in which a patient's heat gained exceeds the patient's heat loss.**

Hyperthermia

❍ **Identify those questions that are important to ask regarding a patient suffering from exposure to the environment.**

What is the source of their exposure? What particular environment were they in? Have they experienced any loss of consciousness? What effects are they feeling in their body?

❍ **Infants and young children are at great risk of generalized hypothermia. What factors increase their risk?**

Infants and young children are small with large surface areas. Their small muscle mass does not allow adequate shivering in children, and none at all in infants. They have less body fat to insulate them from the environment. Younger children need help to protect themselves. They are unable to put on or take off their clothes, which afford them protection in a given environment.

○   **Identify the signs and symptoms of generalized hypothermia and how you would assess a patient experiencing hypothermia.**

Cold or cool skin temperature. Place the back of his hand between the clothing and the patient's abdomen to assess the general temperature of the patient. The patient experiencing a generalized cold emergency will present with cold abdominal skin temperature; a decreasing mental status or motor function, which directly correlates with a degree of hypothermia.

○   **Identify the respiratory variations that may be seen in both the early and late hypothermic patient.**

A patient suffering from early signs of hypothermia will experience rapid breathing. Patients suffering from late hypothermia may experience shallow, slow, or even absent breathing.

○   **A patient experiencing hypothermia will show variances in their pulse rate depending on the severity of the hypothermia. Describe these changes.**

A patient experiencing early hypothermia will have a rapid pulse rate. A patient suffering from late hypothermia may experience a slow, barely palpable, and/or irregular or completely absent pulse rate. Additionally, they may also have a low to absent blood pressure.

○   **Describe the skin of a patient suffering from hypothermia.**

A patient suffering from hypothermia may exhibit skin that is both red in the early stages of hypothermia and, as hypothermia progresses, the skin will become pale, even cyanotic. Its texture may also become stiff and hard.

○   **Identify the appropriate medical care for patients suffering from generalized hypothermia.**

Remove the patient from the environment. Protect the patient from further heat loss. Place in a warm environment as soon as possible. Remove all wet clothing and cover with a blanket. Handle the patient extremely gently. Avoid rough handling of any kind. Do not allow the patient to walk or exert himself or herself in any fashion. Administer oxygen if not already done as part of the initial assessment. Oxygen administered should be warmed and humidified if possible. Assess pulses for 30-45 seconds before starting CPR, as the patient may be bradycardic. The 30 or 40 seconds ensures a good time frame for assessing pulses. If the patient is alert and responding appropriately, actively rewarm the patient with warm blankets, heat packs or hot water bottles to the groin, axillary, and cervical regions. If possible, turn up the heat in the patient compartment of the ambulance.

❍   **You must be able to provide proper emergency medical care for a patient suffering from localized cold injuries. Identify the proper emergency medical care.**

Remove the patient from the environment immediately. Protect the cold injured extremity from further injury. Administer oxygen, if not already done as part of the initial assessment. Remove all wet or restrictive clothing. If it is an early or superficial injury, splint the extremity, cover the extremity, and do not rub it. Do not re-expose to the cold. If it is a late or deep cold injury, remove all jewelry and cover with dry clothing or dressings. Do not break any blisters, rub, or massage the area, apply heat directly to the tissue or attempt to re-warm. Do not allow the patient to walk on any of the affected extremities. When an extremely long or delayed transport is inevitable, then active rapid re-warming should be done.

❍   **List the proper procedure for active rapid re-warming.**

Immerse the affected part in warm water bath.
Monitor the water to ensure that it does not cool from the frozen part.
Continuously stir the water to keep it moving.
Continue until the part is soft and color and sensation return.
Dress the area with a dry sterile dressing.
If it is a hand or a foot, place a dry sterile dressing between fingers and toes.
Protect against re-freezing of the warmed part and expect the patient to complain of severe pain.

❍   **Give an example of an advanced directive.**

Do Not Resuscitate (DNR) orders.

❍   **T/F: The patient does not have the right to refuse resuscitative orders.**

False.

❍   **T/F: DNR orders require a written order from a physician.**

True, in most jurisdictions.

❍   **You arrive at the home of a 68 year-old man who presents with a weak, thready pulse and respirations of eight. The wife states she has DNR orders, but she can't find them. What do you do?**

Begin resuscitative efforts.

❍   **In order to obtain expressed consent from a patient, that patient must . . .**

Be of legal age, be able to make rational decisions, and must be informed of the steps of the procedures and all related risks.

❍   **When must you obtain expressed consent from a patient?**

Before rendering treatment to every conscious, mentally competent adult.

❍   **What is implied consent?**

Implied consent is consent assumed from the unconscious patient requiring emergency intervention.

❍   **Upon what assumption is implied consent based?**

On the assumption that the unconscious patient would consent to lifesaving interventions were he or she conscious.

❍   **When does the principle of implied consent apply to children?**

When life-threatening situations exist and the parent or legal guardian is not available for consent.

❍   **When does the principle of implied consent apply to mentally incompetent adults?**

When life-threatening situations exist and the legal guardian is not available for consent.

❍   **What local issues may effect consent for treating children and mentally incompetent adults?**

Emancipation issues, and state regulations regarding the age of minors.

❍   **What is the legal term for unlawfully touching a patient without his or her consent?**

Battery.

❍   **What is the legal term for providing emergency care when the patient does not consent to the treatment?**

Assault.

❍   **T/F: A patient has the right to refuse treatment, even when that treatment may prove lifesaving.**

True.

❍   **Who can refuse treatment or transport?**

Any mentally competent adult, or in the case of a child or mentally incompetent adult, the parent or legal guardian.

❍   **If you have any doubt as to whether you should or should not provide care to a patient, what should you do?**

Err in favor of providing care.

❍   **How can you protect yourself from the legal consequences of patient refusal?**

Ensure that you document fully and accurately.

❍   **T/F: Before leaving the scene of a patient who refuses transport, you should try to persuade the patient to be transported.**

True. Always err on the side of treatment.

❍   **You suspect that your patient is drunk, but he signs the release form and tells you to leave. Are you legally liable if something happens to this patient and why?**

Yes. A patient under the influence of alcohol is not considered competent to refuse treatment.

❍   **Define negligence.**

Negligence is the deviation from the accepted standard of care resulting in further injury to the patient.

❍   **What are the four components of negligence?**

A duty to act
Breach of that duty
Injury or damage was inflicted, either physical or psychological.
The actions of treating individual caused the injury or damage.

❍   **T/F: In order for there to be a duty to act, a contractual or legal obligation must exist.**

True.

❍   **A patient calls for an ambulance, and the dispatcher confirms that an ambulance will be sent. Do the rescuers on the ambulance have an implied or formal duty to act?**

Implied.

❍ **You begin treatment of a patient. Is continuing treatment an implied or formal duty to act?**

Implied.

❍ **You are treating a patient who is tachypneic, with shallow, inadequate respirations. What might you expect to discover when examining his skin?**

The skin may be pale or cyanotic, and cool and clammy.

❍ **You are called to the home of a three year-old girl. The parents state it has been increasingly difficult to breathe over the past few hours, and she has used her inhaler five times. What might you expect to see on inspection of her chest and belly?**

There may be retractions above the clavicles, between the ribs and below the rib cage. "Seesaw" or paradoxical breathing may be present, where the abdomen and chest move in opposite directions.

❍ **In reference to the case above, what might you expect to see when inspecting her face?**

Nasal flaring may be present. Mucous membranes may be pale or cyanotic. Skin may be cool and diaphoretic. The patient may appear anxious.

❍ **Why is it easier for a child's airway to become obstructed than an adult's airway?**

All structures are smaller and more easily obstructed.

❍ **How does the pharynx in an adult and child differ?**

Infant and children's tongues take up proportionally more space in the mouth than adults do.

❍ **How does the trachea in an adult and child differ?**

Infants and children have narrower tracheas that are obstructed more easily by swelling, and the trachea is also softer and more flexible. The cricoid cartilage is less developed and less rigid, and is the narrowest portion of the child's airway.

❍ **What is the principal difference in the way children and adults breathe?**

The chest wall of the child is softer and the muscles less well developed. Therefore, infants and children rely more heavily on the diaphragm for breathing than adults.

❍   Upon arrival at a motor vehicle crash, you find a woman in her twenties, supine on the street. How do you initially assess circulation?

Palpate the carotid artery.

❍   When using one hand to secure a mask for ventilation, which fingers hold the mask down?

The thumb and index fingers.

❍   What is the purpose of the oxygen reservoir?

The oxygen reservoir allows for a higher concentration of oxygen.

❍   What sizes of masks should you carry for the bag-valve-mask?

Infant, child and adult.

❍   Where should you position the apex of the mask of the bag-valve-mask?

Over the patient's nose.

❍   T/F: Two rescuers using the bag-valve-mask will be more effective than one.

True.

❍   T/F: Position self at the side of the patient's head for optimal performance.

False. You should be positioned at the top of the patient's head.

❍   What adjunctive airways may be necessary to effectively ventilate with the bag-valve-mask?

Oropharyngeal or nasopharyngeal airways.

❍   What characteristics should the self-refilling bag have?

It should be able to be easily cleaned and sterilized.

❍   What kind of valve should the bag-valve-mask have?

A non-jam valve that allows a maximum of oxygen inlet flow of 15L/min.

❍   How often should you repeat ventilations on an adult?

Every five seconds.

○   **How often should you repeat ventilations on a child?**

Every three seconds.

○   **If while ventilating a patient the chest does not rise and fall, what is the first thing you should do?**

Reposition the head.

○   **If while ventilating a patient the chest does not rise and fall, what should you do after repositioning the head?**

If air is escaping from under the mask, reposition fingers and mask.

○   **If while ventilating a patient the chest does not rise and fall, what should you do after repositioning fingers and mask?**

Check for obstruction.

○   **If while ventilating a patient the chest does not rise and fall, what should you do after checking for obstruction?**

Use alternative method of artificial ventilation, e.g. pocket mask, manually triggered device. If necessary, consider the use of adjuncts such as oral or nasal airways.

○   **What precautions should you take in ventilating a patient with suspected trauma or neck injury?**

Immobilize the head and neck. Have an assistant immobilize, or immobilize between your knees.

○   **What type of ventilatory device is contraindicated in children?**

Oxygen powered ventilation devices.

○   **What peak flow rate and percent of oxygen should a flow-restricted oxygen-powered ventilation device be capable of delivering?**

100% at up to 40L/min.

○   **At what pressure should the inspiratory pressure relief valve activate on a flow-restricted oxygen-powered ventilation device?**

60 cc/water.

○   **In addition to a pressure relief valve, what safety features should a flow-restricted oxygen-powered ventilation device have?**

An audible alarm that sounds whenever the relief-valve pressure is exceeded.

○   **How should the trigger be positioned on a flow-restricted oxygen-powered ventilation device?**

In such a way that both hands of the EMT can remain on the mask to hold it in position.

○   **What is a tracheostomy?**

A permanent artificial opening in the trachea.

○   **What special procedures do you need to use when ventilating a tracheostomy patient?**

If unable to artificially ventilate, try suction, then artificial ventilation through the nose and mouth; sealing the stoma may improve ability to artificially ventilate from above or may clear obstruction. You need to seal the mouth and nose when air is escaping.

PHARMACOLOGY

Drug	Dose
Epinephrine	1 mg of 1:10,000 solution IV or 2-2.5 mg down ETT Q 3-5 minutes
Atropine	0.5-1 mg IV or down ETT Q 5 minutes up to 3 mg total
Lidocaine	1.0-1.5 mg/kg IV bolus, followed by 2-4 mg IV infusion, 0.5 mg/kg IV repeat bolus after 10 minutes. If ventricular ectopy persists, repeat 0.5-0.75 mg/kg IV bolus up to max total dose of 3 mg/kg.
Vasopressin	40 Units IVP (one time dose) for shock-refractory VF. (Must wait 10 minutes after vasopressin before administering dose of epinephrine).
Procainamide	20-30 mg/min for total loading dose of 17 mg/kg or until QRS widened by 50% or arrhythmia is suppressed. 20-50 mg/ min IV infusion for recurrent VF/VT
Amiodarone	300 mg IVP, followed by 150 mg IVP Q 3-5 minutes for refractory ventricular fibrillation/pulseless ventricular tachycardia (VF/VT). 150 mg IVP over 10 minutes for stable monomorphic or polymorphic VT. Maximum total IV dose for 24 hours not to exceed 2.2 grams.
Verapamil	2.5-5 mg IV bolus over 1-2 minutes, may repeat with 5-10 mg IV Q 15 minutes until max dose of 30 mg.
Diltiazem	0.25 mg/kg IV bolus over 2 minutes, followed by infusion of 5-15 mg/hr. May repeat bolus of 0.35 mg/kg if heart rate control not achieved.
Adenosine	6 mg IV rapid bolus over 1-3 seconds, followed by IV bolus of normal saline. Elevate the extremity. If no response after 1-2 minutes, 12 mg repeat IV bolus. If still no response after another 1-2 minutes, can give third dose of 12 mg IVP.
Magnesium Sulfate	1-2 grams IV over 1-2 minutes

Sodium Bicarbonate   1 mEq/kg IV bolus, followed by 0.5 mEq IV Q 10 minutes

Morphine   1-3 mg slow IV push

Calcium Chloride   8-16 mg/kg of 10% solution or 10 ml prefilled syringe IV, may
                     repeat at 10 minute intervals if needed.

Dopamine   2-20 mcg/kg/min IV infusion. 2-5 mcg/kg/min=dopaminergic,
                     5-10 beta, 10-20 alpha

Dobutamine   2.5-15 mcg/kg/min IV infusion

Isoproterenol   2-10 mcg/min IV infusion

Inamrinone   0.75 mg/kg IV over 10-15 minutes, followed by 2-5 mcg/kg/min
                     infusion.

Norepinephrine   4 mcg/min infusion

Nitroprusside   0.5-8.0 mcg/kg/min infusion, titrated to desired blood pressure.

Nitroglycerin   For angina- 0.3 to 0.4 mg sublingual, may be repeated Q 5 minutes
                     For unstable angina-12.5-25 mcg IV bolus, followed by infusion
                         of 10-20 mcg/min, increased by 5-10 mcg/min every 5-10
                         minutes until desired hemodynamic response or
                         termination of chest pain is achieved.

Metoprolol   5 mg IV bolus Q 5 minutes to a total of 15 mg or until heart rate
                         Drops between 50-60/min. Then start oral dose of 50 mg
                         Twice daily for 24 hours, increased to 100 mg BID.

Atenolol   5 mg IV over 5 minutes, followed by second dose of 5 mg IV after
                         10 minutes. Then start oral dose of 50 mg BID if tolerated.

Propranolol   1-3 mg IV over 2-5 minutes, not to exceed 1 mg/min, repeat after
                         2 minutes to a total dose of 0.1 mg/kg.

Esmolol   Loading dose of 250-500 mcg/kg IV for 1 minute, followed by
                         maintenance infusion of 25-50 mcg/kg/min for 4 minutes,
                         titrated upward by 25-50 mcg/kg per minute at 5-10
                         minute intervals to a maximum dose of 300 mcg/kg/min.

Labetolol   10 mg IVP over 1-2 minutes, may repeat or double dose every 10
                         minutes up to maximum total dose of 150 mg.

Furosemide   20-80 mg IV bolus over 1-2 minutes

Streptokinase   1.5 million units IV over 30-60 minutes

r-TPA (Alteplase)   15 mg IV bolus over 1 minute, followed by 0.75 mg/kg IV infusion
                       over 30 minutes (not to exceed 50 mg), followed by 0.50
                       mg/kg IV infusion over next 60 minutes (not to exceed 35
                       mg).

Anistreplase (APSAC) 30 units IV bolus over 5 minutes

ALGORITHM PROTOCOLS

Basic Life Support

All cases: Two initial breaths, then CPR compressions at rate of 80-100 per minute
One rescuer: 15:2 ratio of compressions to ventilations
Two rescuer or Pediatric: 5:1 ratio of compressions to ventilations.

Ventricular Fibrillation, or Pulseless Ventricular Tachycardia

CPR until defibrillator ready
Defibrillate 200 J, check pulse and rhythm
Defibrillate 200-300 J, check pulse and rhythm
Defibrillate 360 J, check pulse and rhythm
Intubate, IV access
Epinephrine 1 mg IV/2-2.5 mg down ETT Q 3-5 minutes
Defibrillate 360 J after each drug dose
Options:
Lidocaine 1.5 mg IV Q 3-5 minutes to max dose of 3 mg/kg
Amiodarone 300 mg IVP, 150 mg IVP Q 3-5 minutes
Magnesium 1-2 grams IV
Procainamide 30 mg/min IV to max total dose of 17 mg/kg
Sodium Bicarbonate 1 mEq/kg IV

Stable Ventricular Tachycardia

Airway, IV access, Oxygen
Lidocaine 1-1.5 mg/kg IV bolus
Lidocaine 0.5-0.75 mg/kg IV Q 5-10 minutes to total of 3 mg/kg, or
Procainamide 20-30 mg/min to maximum of 17 mg/kg, or
Amiodarone 150 mg IVP over 10 minutes, may repeat Q 10 minutes as needed, or
Consider synchronized cardioversion

Stable Wide-Complex Tachycardia

Airway, IV access, Oxygen
Lidocaine 1-1.5 mg/kg IV bolus
Lidocaine 0.5-0.75 mg/kg IV Q 5-10 minutes to total of 3 mg/kg
Adenosine 6 mg rapid IV bolus, wait 1-2 minutes. If no response,
Adenosine 12 mg rapid IV bolus, wait 1-2 minutes, or
Procainamide 20-30 mg/min to maximum of 17 mg/kg (for normal LVEF), or
Amiodarone 150 mg IVP over 10 minutes, may repeat every 10 minutes as needed, or
Consider synchronized cardioversion

Pulseless Electrical Activity (PEA) or (EMD)

CPR, intubate, IV access

Consider hypovolemia, hypoxia, cardiac tamponade, tension pneumothorax, hypothermia, massive PE, drug overdose, hyperkalemia, acidosis, massive MI

Epinephrine 1 mg IV/ETT Q 3-5 minutes

Atropine 1 mg IV bolus if heart rate < 60/min.

Asystole

CPR, intubate, IV access

Confirm asystole in at least two leads

Consider hypoxia, hypothermia, drug overdose, hyperkalemia, hypokalemia.

Consider external pacing

Epinephrine 1 mg IV/ETT Q 3-5 minutes

Atropine 1 mg IV/ETT, repeat in 3-5 minutes

Bradycardia (< 60/min), symptomatic

Airway, IV access, Oxygen

Atropine 0.5-1 mg IV bolus Q 3-5 minutes up to 2-3 mg total

External pacemaker

Options:

Dopamine 5-20 mcg/kg/min

Epinephrine 2-10 mcg/min

Consider Isoproterenol

Unstable Tachycardia (> 150/min)

Airway, IV access, Oxygen

Synchronized cardioversion 100 J

Synchronized cardioversion 200 J

Synchronized cardioversion 300 J

Synchronized cardioversion 360 J

Consider trial of medicines for wide-complex tachycardia algorhythm

Stable PSVT

Airway, IV access, Oxygen

Vagal maneuvers

Adenosine 6 mg rapid IV bolus, wait 1-2 minutes

Adenosine 12 mg rapid IV bolus, wait 1-2 minutes

Adenosine 18 mg rapid IV bolus, wait 1-2 minutes

If narrow complex, consider verapamil, digoxin, beta-blockers or diltiazem

If wide complex, consider lidocaine or procainamide

Consider synchronized cardioversion

BIBLIOGRAPHY

Braunwald, E., Heart Disease: A Textbook of Cardiovascular Medicine, (6th Edition), W. B. Saunders Co., 2001.

Cummins, Richard O., Advanced Cardiac Life Support, American Heart Association, ISBN 0-87493-327-7, 2003.

Fuster, V., Ross, R., Topol, E., Atherosclerosis and Coronary Artery Disease, (2nd Edition) Lippincott, Williams & Wilkins, 2004.

Kaplan, N., Lieberman, E., Clinical Hypertension, (8th Edition), Lippincott, Williams & Wilkins, 2002.

Podrid, P., Kowey, P., Cardiac Arrhythmia: Mechanisms, Diagnosis, and Management, (2nd Edition) Lippincott, Williams & Wilkins, 2001.

Popma, J., Leon, M., Topol, E., Atlas of Interventional Cardiology, (2nd Edition) W. B. Saunders Co., 2003.

Topol, E., Califf, R., Isner, J., Textbook of Cardiovascular Medicine, (2nd Edition) Lippincott, Williams & Wilkins, 2002.

Wagner, G., Marriott, H. J. L., Marriotts Practical Electrocardiography, (10th Edition), Lippincott, Williams & Wilkins, 2001.

Willerson, J., Cohn, J., Cardiovascular Medicine, (2nd Edition) Churchill Livingstone, 2000.

Zipes, D., Jalife, J., Cardiac Electrophysiology: From Cell to Bedside, (4th Edition), W. B. Saunders Co., 2004.